THE CUCUMBER DIET™

The Power of Conscious Eating

Copyright © 2019 Jay Arnold

Gracious contributors: W. Scott Deaver, Maria Pfeffer, Bruce Campbell, Robb Soslow, Frank Lomento.
Book design Ryan Currier, Food Photography Kaz Weida.
Cover design James L. Lewis, Cover Photography Alexander Newman.

TM - Trademark 2019 The Cucumber Diet, LLC

Cucumber Diet:

A Path To Conscious Eating

Introduction

Welcome to Cucumber Club...
"Is this your first time?"
"Yes, I'm a newcumber ..."

Growing up, I was a small, skinny kid. I ate what I wanted with the only stipulation being that it tasted good. We were taught to clean our plates, encouraged to eat until we felt full. And asking for seconds was considered polite. We ate a lot of red meat, some chicken, and very little fish—usually in the form of flounder. As a kid, flounder was universally considered punishment food. Somehow, even steeped in butter, it was cringe-worthy. My mother served reasonable portions, and there was little conversation about what was or wasn't good for you – just what tasted good.

Liver was the only exception. We were told the high iron in liver was good for us, but I don't think anyone bought the story. We held our noses and ate it anyway. Except me, of course. I actually liked the stuff. Years later, liver would be cast aside, deemed too high in cholesterol to be healthy. The healthy liver was now nasty liver? I was unsettled by the idea that something once considered wholesome could suddenly become unhealthy. Confusion sets in.

It wasn't until 1969 that the White House Conference on Food, Nutrition, and Health made a recommendation to FDA to develop a structure for identifying nutritional attributes of food[1]. And it would take until 1973 before any regulations were put in place by the FDA.

FDA-regulated foods were required to include the total number of calories, protein, carbohydrate, and fat. Also included were the percentages of the U.S. Recommended Daily Allowance (RDA) of protein, vitamins A and C, thiamin, riboflavin, niacin, calcium, and iron. If you believe it, sodium, saturated fatty acids, and polyunsaturated fatty acids were added "at the manufacturer's discretion.[2]" The conversation about what was healthy and unhealthy was just getting started, but by then, many of us were set in our ways.

What a surprise to find the healthy tomato juice we drank was serving up an entire day's worth of sodium. Then came the proliferation of unhealthy, highly processed foods. Margarine, artificial sweeteners, and the now-infamous red dye #2 sparked a sense of awareness that our diets were deeply compromised.

Then in 1992 (this wasn't even our idea, Sweden developed and published it almost twenty years prior), guidance arrived in the form of the "Food Pyramid.[3]" In 2005, the Pyramid was updated to reflect our changing ideas about nutrition. By 2011, however, the Food Pyramid was scrapped altogether and replaced with MyPlate. MyPlate reflected an effort to curb carb consumption, flipping the spot grains had formerly occupied with vegetables. We had been advised as part of the Food Pyramid to consume 6-11 servings of breads and grains daily. Under My Plate that amount dropped dramatically to only 30% of our totally daily intake.

This growing awareness of the dangers of things we had previously seen as healthy, like fluffy, processed white bread, was a difficult adjustment. Eat bread. No, don't eat bread. Nobody seemed to have a clear answer.

And then the new trend became clear. It's fat and cholesterol that are unhealthy! Got it. So I leaned into foods billed as "healthy", "light" or "low fat". But as it turns out, those were all heavily processed, and in turn, not so healthy at all. Worse yet, I had no idea that these "healthy" processed foods were loaded with sugar, among other things, which made them, you guessed it, fattening.

And as a result, I gained weight. So, I did what you're supposed to do. I ate less. I went to the gym and worked out regularly. It was hard and I was miserable, but I managed to take off about half the weight I had gained in the process.

Over the course of the next decade, however, I slowly gained the weight back. Not at once, just a pound or two a year. While it didn't seem like a lot along the way – it added up. I'm sure it's a story that sounds familiar.

I was frustrated. I'd worked in the weight loss industry for years, read a ton on the topic, and been to spas and clinics. I reasoned I had to know enough to figure out how to eat healthy, be satisfied and keep my weight in check. What I discovered is that I was eating all wrong. Low fat processed foods were not the answer. After a few dead ends and wrong turns, I found the right path for me. And it worked better than I ever expected. Although at the time, I didn't think about the solution I'd discovered as a diet. And yet here we are.

1 Mayer, Jean. "A REPORT ON THE WHITE HOUSE CONFERENCE ON FOOD, NUTRITION AND HEALTH - Mayer - 1969 - Nutrition Reviews - Wiley Online Library." Nutrition Reviews, John Wiley & Sons, Ltd (10.1111), 27 Apr. 2009, https://onlinelibrary.wiley.com/doi/abs/10.1111/j.1753-4887.1969.tb06449.x

2 Institute of Medicine (US) Committee on Examination of Front-of-Package Nutrition Rating Systems and Symbols. "History of Nutrition Labeling." Front-of-Package Nutrition Rating Systems and Symbols: Phase I Report., U.S. National Library of Medicine, 1 Jan. 1970, https://www.ncbi.nlm.nih.gov/books/NBK209859/

3 "A Brief History of USDA Food Guides." Choose MyPlate, 30 Nov. 2018, https://www.choosemyplate.gov/brief-history-usda-food-guides

The Cucumber Diet and The Art of Conscious Eating

Oddly it started with watermelon. I noticed watermelon filled me up but because it was so sweet, I thought it had to have a ton of calories. Imagine my surprise discovering watermelon was only 30 calories a serving. A watermelon serving is ¾ of a cup, so even if you have four servings it's still only 120 calories. That's pretty much an entire plate of watermelon. I soon discovered there are a lot of other foods just like watermelon and they're known as low-calorie-density foods. And yes, you guessed it, cucumbers are among them.

For all the right reasons, as you will discover, cucumbers were the perfect way to lean into a diet that can become a lifestyle. A lifestyle of conscious eating filled with delicious, clean, healthy, satisfying foods.

Conscious eating is really so simple. It's just that nobody taught us how to do it. Until now.

Why Cucumbers?

What did the cucumber say to the tomato?
Say what you like, I've got thick skin.

Since I'm reasonably certain The Cucumber Diet will seem like an odd name for a diet, let's talk about cucumbers. To start, cucumbers are delicious and versatile. Refreshing, crisp and bulky they rank in the top ten most popular veggies for a reason.

While there are many exciting benefits to this remarkable super-food, cucumbers are also an effective way to introduce the benefits of low-calorie density (LCD) foods. We'll get into that later, but read on. There's a lot more to get excited about other than learning cucumbers are actually a fruit. Yep, a fruit! You heard that right. However, like tomatoes, most people still classify cucumbers as vegetables.

There's a world of whole foods to choose from, so you're probably asking yourself why cucumbers are the star of this show. These unassuming, crisply translucent green veggies once tossed onto salads as an afterthought are a powerhouse of nutrients that deserve to be center stage. Take your pick of any of the following reasons to justifying adding cucumbers into any and every meal.

Cucumbers are low-calorie dense food.

We'll cover exactly why low-calorie-density foods are so powerful later, but cucumbers definitely fit the bill. They give you a lot of nutritional bang for the caloric cost. Each cup of cucumbers is less than 20 calories, and an entire 11-ounce cucumber contains only 45.[4] That means you can pack away an entire bowl of cucumbers without guilt, making them a fantastic foundation for healthy, filling meals. And another advantage to whole foods like cucumbers is that you get the benefits of the nutrients without worrying about the side effects of additives.

Cucumbers also boast a high-water count, which makes them particularly well suited for weight loss. Thirteen different studies found that people who consumed foods with high water content and a low-calorie count saw a significant decrease in body weight.[5]

Cucumbers are packed with antioxidants & anti-inflammatories.

Studies indicate the nutrients in cucumbers may tackle inflammation by blocking a group of enzymes called matrix metalloproteinase. These enzymes are implicated in arthritis, chronic inflammation, and wrinkle formation.[6]

Cucumbers also contain fisetin, a dietary flavonoid that studies indicate may reduce the risk of breast, ovarian, and other types of cancer.[7]

Cucumbers may help regulate blood sugar.

Eating whole foods helps avoid the high-sugar and fat content of junk food that can lead to diabetes and heart disease, but cucumbers take it up a notch. Several studies indicate cucumbers may play an important role in regulating blood sugar and reducing complications from Type II diabetes.[8]

Cucumbers promote brain health.

The ability of cucumbers to promote cognitive function comes from the same dietary flavonoid we mentioned earlier—fisetin. The results in some studies suggest fisetin may support brain health in people with Alzheimer's and help prevent or delay the impact of age-related neurological diseases.[9]

Cucumbers support bone health.

It's not just calcium that builds healthy bones. Vitamin K is also an essential component of bone health, and low levels can lead to increased bone fractures and a higher risk of osteoporosis.[10] Having just one cup of unpeeled cucumbers will provide over 20 percent of the recommended daily value of vitamin K.

Cucumbers keep you hydrated.

Have you ever bitten into a cucumber and felt the crisp, cool gush of all that nutrient-rich water across your tongue? The importance of water cannot be overstated, both in terms of health and weight loss. Dehydration can affect physical performance, processing speed, metabolic speed, and overall bodily health. Cucumbers have a water content of 95.2% water, so even a meager 5-ounce serving provides more than 25% of your suggested daily water intake.

As you can see, there are quite a few reasons to make cucumbers the centerpiece of any weight loss plan, or really any healthy diet. For the

Cucumber Diet, we recommend using organic or hydroponic cucumbers. Whether you have access to a farmer's market or a chain supermarket, fresh, local cucumbers provide a superior taste to really sink your teeth into.

4 Self Nutrition Data, "Cucumber with peel, raw, Nutrition Facts and Calories"

5 Stelmach-Mardas, Marta, et al. "Link between Food Energy Density and Body Weight Changes in Obese Adults." Nutrients, MDPI, 20 Apr. 2016, https://www.ncbi.nlm.nih.gov/pmc/articles/PMC4848697/

6 Ríos, J. L., Recio, M. C., Escandell, J. M., & Andújar, I. (2009). Inhibition of transcription factors by plant-derived compounds and their implications in inflammation and cancer. Retrieved from https://www.ncbi.nlm.nih.gov/pubmed/19355962

7 Lall, Rahul K, et al. "Dietary Flavonoid Fisetin for Cancer Prevention and Treatment." Molecular Nutrition & Food Research, U.S. National Library of Medicine, June 2016, https://www.ncbi.nlm.nih.gov/pmc/articles/PMC6261287/ Person. "Why Cucumber Is a Legitimate Super Food." Men's Health, Men's Health, 18 Apr. 2019, https://www.menshealth.com/uk/nutrition/food-drink/a27191434/cucumber-super-food/

8 Dixit, Yamini, and Anand Kar. "Protective Role of Three Vegetable Peels in Alloxan Induced Diabetes Mellitus in Male Mice." Plant Foods for Human Nutrition (Dordrecht, Netherlands), U.S. National Library of Medicine, Sept. 2010, https://www.ncbi.nlm.nih.gov/pubmed/20614191

9 Currais, Antonio, et al. "Modulation of p25 and Inflammatory Pathways by Fisetin Maintains Cognitive Function in Alzheimer's Disease Transgenic Mice." Aging Cell, BlackWell Publishing Ltd, Apr. 2014, http://www.ncbi.nlm.nih.gov/pubmed/24341874

10 LD, Megan Ware RDN. "Vitamin K: Health Benefits, Daily Intake, and Sources." Medical News Today, MediLexicon International, 22 Jan. 2018, https://www.medicalnewstoday.com/articles/219867.php

The ABCs of Conscious Eating

Why did the cucumber blush?
It saw the salad dressing.

The Cucumber Diet is based on the notion of conscious eating. Conscious eating is about being aware. It's a simple, straightforward concept I like to think of as the ABCs of a healthy lifestyle.

Aware of…
  A: **what** you're eating
  B: **how much** you're eating
  C: what each meal **costs** in calories

To simplify the practice of conscious eating, we've broken it down into three principles:
  A: Whole foods and low-calorie-density foods (**what** you're eating)
  B: Serving size (**how much** you're eating)
  C: Do the math (what is the caloric **cost** of each meal)

We'll elaborate on each of these principles in the following chapters. While you'll become more aware of these tenets of conscious eating as you practice them, we've also put a meal plan with a daily caloric allocation in place that's easy to follow. The goal is a lifetime of conscious eating, but we have learned that the easiest way to get there is by following a clear, simple meal plan until you master the concept.

A Calorie-Managed Plan

All meal recipes and options provided as part of the Cucumber Diet are designed to fit perfectly into the daily caloric allocation. The Cucumber Diet is primarily focused on whole and low-calorie-density foods. Food that are higher in fiber and protein, lower in fats and carbohydrates.

There's no starving on this diet. You'll eat four meals a day. The Cucumber Diet uses easy recipes, including grab and go options for every meal so that you can stay on plan even when life throws you a curveball. If you do go off-menu, simply stay within the allocated calories for that meal to make sure you're not exceeding your total daily caloric allocation.

Your daily menu might include:

Breakfast: Sunny-Side Up Avocado Toast (243 calories)

Lunch: The Moroccan Cucumber Bowl (410 calories)

Dinner: Half Cucumber Bowl, (150 calories), Cheddar and Parmesan Risotto (405 calories) (total 555 calories)

Dessert: Oatmeal & Dark Chocolate Chunk Cookies (200 calories)

Caloric cost of this delicious, well-rounded menu? 1,408 calories. The customizable menus of the Cucumber Diet plan give you flexibility to edge up to 1500 calories with some extras like cream in your coffee and still meet your goals.

The customizable menus of the Cucumber Diet plan give you flexibility while still maintaining your total daily caloric allocation. For women, it's 1500 calories a day. For men, the range expands to 1900 calories. Don't worry about counting calories for now, though. Simply follow the plan, and you'll meet the optimal daily caloric allocation.

While we coach you not to focus on calorie counting while on the plan, we do show the calories to help you gain a better awareness of the caloric cost of each meal. Because ultimately, calories matter.

As part of the Cucumber Diet, you'll see grab-n-go options offered for every meal. These choices are designed to help you stay on plan with convenient, off-the-shelf solutions from your local supermarket. We've done our best to give you general guidance about calories for grab-n-go options, but you should also read the labels with special attention to serving sizes.

Cucumber Diet Daily caloric allocations by meal are as follows:

Women

Breakfast: Breakfast offerings or grab-n-go options (250 calories)

Lunch: Select a cucumber bowl recipe OR use the build your own chart (450 calories)

Dinner: A half cucumber bowl (150), accompanied by a dinner selection (500 calories) (total 650 calories)

Dessert: Fruit, quick desserts, grab-n-go or cookies for a crowd (150 calories)

Daily Total: 1500 calories

Men

Breakfast: Breakfast offerings or grab-n-go options (250 calories)

Lunch: Select a cucumber bowl recipe OR build your own (600 calories) *We suggest build your own to meet the caloric allocation for men. If you choose to make one of our recipes double a protein or dairy.

Dinner: A half cucumber bowl (150), accompanied by a dinner selection (750 calories) (total 900 calories) *For men increase the dinner serving size by half, or 1.5 servings.

Dessert: Fruit, quick desserts, grab-n-go or cookies for a crowd (200 calories)

Daily Total: 1900 calories

The average woman needs to eat about 2000 calories per day to maintain, and 1500 calories to lose one pound of weight per week. An average man needs 2500 calories to maintain, and 2000 to lose one pound of weight per week. But everyone's daily caloric needs are different. We'll cover how to determine your individual needs shortly.

The plan also includes unlimited cucumbers, water, and tea so you'll never go hungry (or thirsty). You can also indulge in coffee but sideline the cream and sugar as much as possible. If you must use cream, sugar, or both, choose options that are lighter in calories and be stingy.

Let's Eat

We encourage you to prepare as many meals as you can, but we also know that life happens. Most of us don't have the kind of time it takes to prepare all our meals in advance. With that in mind, in addition to easy, quick recipes, we've included the grab-n-go options you can pick up from your local supermarket.

Breakfast begins with one of fifteen simple recipes. A few of the recipes yield more than one serving, and you'll see that clearly indicated next to the listed calorie count. If you're the kind of person that likes to eat the same meal regularly, look for recipes like garden quinoa cups or cashew apple oatmeal snack cups. We've also included a selection of grab-n-go items for when you're running late or missed your alarm. (Hey, it happens.)

Lunch features one of our signature cucumber bowls. They're delicious, fast, and flexible. You can choose one of our eight cucumber bowl recipes, or build your own cucumber bowl using the handy build-your-own chart. Be as adventurous as you like with the broad range of ingredients that you can mix and match to suit your taste. On average, it takes less than ten minutes to make a delicious cucumber bowl.

Dinner begins with a smaller, half Cucumber Bowl. For your main course, there are fifteen fantastic recipes that run the gamut from seafood to vegetarian. All recipes serve a family size of 4 and most meals can be on the table in 20-30 minutes or less. For nights when you're too overwhelmed to cook, you'll also find a selection of grab-n-go items to suit almost any taste

Got a sweet tooth? You're in good company. We saved the best for last with a range of desserts that can be as simple as a wedge of salted melon or as indulgent as oatmeal chocolate cookies. You can also stock up on some of our grab-n-go suggestions and keep them in the pantry for when you're in a pinch

The "A" of Conscious Eating: Low-Calorie-Density and the Whole Foods Advantage

Where do cucumbers go for a date?
The salad bar.

When we talk about whole foods, we're not suggesting you shop at a certain well-known health food store chain. What the Cucumber Diet advocates, however, is the use of whole foods, or foods that are as close to their natural state as possible. It's the difference between eating veggies and veggie chips or eating apples vs. applesauce.

The Cucumber Diet does not, however, assume you will eat 100% whole foods. While that would be ideal, it's not practical. Of course, "minimally processed foods" are better than heavily processed foods and convenient, reasonable solutions. But every once in a while, a processed chip or a bit of junk food will call your name. Have it, don't deprive yourself. Simply eat processed foods in moderation, better yet accompany your treat with a whole food for balance.

Whole foods do not need to be strictly organic or local. Their value lies in the fact that they have not been processed and thus maintain their original nutrient value and benefits. And they let you avoid the unhealthy additives that many processed foods employ.

So, one advantage of filling up on whole foods is that it naturally curbs your consumption of processed foods, which can be high in salt, fat, and sugar. Eating more whole foods aids in weight loss, and diets high in vegetables, fruits, and whole grains are linked to lower rates of heart disease, cancer, and diabetes.[11] Many whole foods, especially fruits and vegetables, contain natural compounds called phytochemicals, which can act as antioxidants.

A combination of whole foods can also be critical for nutrient absorption and the increased fiber that aids digestion. Ingredients of recipes made with whole foods create a sort of synergy, with nutrients working in concert to boost the absorption of vitamins or minerals. That's why the bit of fat in a simple vinegar and oil-based dressing on your cucumber bowl can increase the nutrient value of all those veggies and fruits you consume.

It's like the difference between filling up the gas tank in your high-performance sports car with regular unleaded versus racing fuel. Whole foods are like racing fuel, optimized for your engine and the perfect mixture for proper combustion and energy production.

Why are whole foods crucial to any weight loss plan?

Processed foods tend to be high in salt, fat, and sugar, while whole foods are unprocessed and lower in sugar. The lower sugar content means that not only are you saving your caloric intake for substance instead of fluff, but you'll avoid the blood sugar slumps between meals that can drive overeating.[12]

Whole foods are also higher in fiber.

Fruits and vegetables and whole grains all have one thing in common. They're an excellent source of fiber in your diet. More fiber intake can not only make you feel fuller and less likely to snack, but it can improve your gut health and overall nutrient absorption.[13]

While the importance of whole foods can't be overstated, we also need to include another critical component of what makes a successful weight loss strategy—low-calorie-density foods.

Low-Calorie-Density (LCD): The Better Deal

Not all foods are created equal. For the purpose of weight loss, you'll want to consume low-calorie dense, whole foods. Low-calorie density refers to the energy or caloric density of a food. For instance, vegetables like cucumbers have about 30 calories per 100 grams versus chocolate, which has 550 calories in 100 grams. The low-calorie dense, high-water content of cucumbers makes them an ideal food to jump start weight loss.

In a nutshell, low-calorie-density foods are more food for fewer calories.

In contrast, high-calorie density foods are those that offer less food at a higher caloric cost. Take for example that delicious, dense cheesecake that is your favorite go-to dessert. A few forkfuls are nothing to worry about, but most of us don't stop there. An entire slice of cheesecake is a high-density concoction rich in eggs, cheese, cream, and plenty of carbs that will set you back more than 400 calories. In contrast, an entire plate full of low-density berries topped with two tablespoons of ricotta and a dash of cocoa will tip the scales at just under 150 calories. And with fruit you get the bonus of fiber, which is likely to leave you feeling full and energized after dinner rather than bloated.

It's a rather simple equation.

Low-calorie density = more food less calories

High density foods = less food more calories

Studies confirm those who consume low-calorie dense diets eat fewer total calories per day. Lower calorie consumption is linked to reduced body weight and BMI as well as smaller waist circumference.[14] In fact, focus on consuming lower-calorie dense foods coupled with reducing fat intake can be a more effective weight loss strategy than a low-fat diet on its own.[15] Experts speculate this is because fibrous fruits and vegetables are more filling and reduce hunger while simultaneously increasing nutrient absorption.

Here's a list of some low-calorie density foods you'll want to incorporate more of in your diet on the following page.

Vegetables

Asparagus - Beetroot - Broccoli - Cabbage - Cauliflower
Celery - Cucumbers - Garlic - Green Beans - Lettuce
Onion - Radish - Spinach - Zucchini

Fruits

Apples - Blueberries - Cantaloupe - Honeydew - Mango
Orange - Peach - Pineapple - Watermelon

Protein

Turkey - Chicken Breast - Cod - Tilapia - Egg Whites

Starches

Boiled Potatoes - Brown Rice - Oatmeal Beans

It's also worth noting that low-calorie dense whole foods tend to cost less, primarily because you're not paying for production expenses. Foods that can go from farm to table can cut out the factory and packaging costs. While they may take you a little longer to wash, cut, and prepare, whole foods also give you the time to focus on being intentional about what you eat.

By doing a little prep work, you'll find yourself with a few extra minutes as you stir or chop to think about what you're about to eat. This paradigm shift of slowing down and engaging in conscious eating is the kind of habit that makes the Cucumber Diet more than a weight loss plan. It's a catalyst that can change the way you nourish yourself and your loved ones.

The "B" of Conscious Eating:
Serving Size Matters

Why did the cucumber cross the street?
Because it was green.

As children, we're taught to clean our plates and eat until we feel full. Meantime, serving sizes at most restaurants have ballooned into meals that tip the scales of our entire daily caloric allocation in one sitting. This also directly impacts our perception of what a proper serving size looks like.

Dinner Plates

In the 60's the average dinner plate was between 7 and 9 inches. Today, the average size of a dinner plate is between 11 and 12 inches.[16] Many restaurants go up to an astounding 13 inches. That's a surface increase of over 35%. And of course, we're inclined to fill our plates. Starting to see the problem?

It's not our fault. We're conditioned to eat as much as we can. If you look at a 12-inch plate of food, your mind assumes you need that much food to feel satisfied. Visually, our perceptions of what a proper serving size looks like are dramatically skewed.

Interestingly, in a new study by the International Journal of Obesity, researchers determined participants consumed 92%, on average, of what was before them.[17] Naturally, larger plates mean larger serving sizes. However, if you decrease the size of your plate to 9 inches from 12 inches, you would reduce your serving size about 20%, and consequently consume 20% fewer calories. That would make a big difference in your daily caloric cost and snowball into increased weight loss over time. Every little bit counts.

Decreasing plate size is an easy first step in getting back to basics on serving size. If you can, switch to a salad plate but pay attention to how that changes your consumption. If you find yourself justifying going back for seconds, upgrade to a slightly larger plate that will help you feel full.

How Does that Serving Size Look?

Let's use something basic, like cereal. Of course, no two portions of cereal are alike. A serving of Corn Flakes, which is not very dense due to their shape and consistency, is one cup. A serving size of something very dense and compact like granola may only be ½ a cup.

Try this experiment to test your sense of serving sizes. Pour the amount of cereal you would normally eat into your bowl and set that aside. It's likely that, like most of us, you use the free pour method where you eyeball the serving size based on your bowl. Then take a measuring cup and measure one serving size according to the packaging instructions, which will likely be between ½ and a whole cup. Then pour that into another bowl of the same size and compare the two. It's likely that the unmeasured portion you eyeballed is going to be much more than one serving. Seeing what a single serving looks like in your own bowl can be staggering, but it gives you a better sense of what a reasonable serving looks like. Repeat this with several items you normally eat using your own bowls and plates.

Assessing Serving Sizes

Since most of the foods the Cucumber Diet promotes are whole foods and low-calorie-density foods, serving size will be less of a concern. Whole foods are not processed and have fewer sugars and other fattening junk. In most cases, you'll eat more food for fewer calories. But with most other foods, serving size matters, particularly when it comes to proteins and fats.

When you go to a restaurant, you can expect to get a much larger serving size than appropriate. A reasonable serving size for proteins like fish, steak, or chicken should be between two and four ounces. Most restaurants will serve between eight and twelve-ounces. It costs very little to increase serving size and since customers often balk at the cost when served smaller portions, restaurants will simply add more to avoid criticisms about value.

At home, it's easier to measure out two to four ounces, but at a restaurant, you don't have that option. I do one of two things when eating out. I'm not shy about sharing, and if someone is willing to split an entrée, bingo. That's half the serving size. When you order, you can also ask the waiter to put half your portion in a take-out container and put it aside. Get it off your plate, and your mind will adapt to the serving size in front of you. It still doesn't mean you need to finish your plate, but at least you're getting close to appropriate serving size. That's conscious eating.

Measuring is not a bad thing, either. And you don't necessarily need to measure every time. Practicing measurement in the beginning will give you a realistic visual of an appropriate serving size. Once it's become a habit, you'll automatically be able to eyeball and eat appropriate serving sizes.

Slow Down

Slowing down isn't a new idea. You've heard before that it takes 20 minutes to feel full once you start eating. If that's true, you may spend as many as fifteen minutes eating beyond your capacity or your hunger. This is why after finishing a large meal, we often feel exhausted and "stuffed." We simply keep eating until we found the bottom of the bowl, no matter the caloric cost.

We often rush. In a society where we're conditioned to get it done, it feels natural to unconsciously shovel food into our mouths. This frantic pace of consumption makes it harder to digest, and many times we barely know what we ate. Slowing down allows you to enjoy your meal and feel satisfied before you're done eating. Practicing conscious eating makes you less likely to clean your plate, particularly if you're feeling satisfied before you finish.

One way you can practice this tenet of conscious eating is simple. **Put down your fork after every bite.**

Most of us don't think about it, but we are much too efficient in moving food from plate to mouth. Try it and see. Putting your fork down after every bite slows your eating and allows you to experience the pleasure of food. And you'll eat a little bit less into the bargain.

The "C" of Conscious Eating: Do the Math

Why did the cucumber blush?
It saw the salad dressing

Most of us have no idea how many calories we consume in a day because no one taught us to do the math. It's branded as negative, laborious, or being a "slave to calories." We are programmed to eat until full or until we hit the bottom of the bowl, with little or no awareness of calories.

Being aware of your caloric intake is a tenet of conscious eating. Awareness alone is a valuable tool, and it's a common-sense first step to lifestyle change. How can you manage your weight if you don't know how many calories you're consuming?

Most structured weight loss plans that supply meals encourage us not to bother counting calories. They say "don't weigh this, don't think of measuring that. It's hard. Let us do it for you." Do these types of plans work? Sure they can, but they don't teach you much beyond how to open a box.

These pre-packaged diet plans have a model that encourages dependency instead of self-reliance. While the calories may be pre-counted for you, you're eating highly processed foods filled with a litany of chemical additives. Take a glance at the labels and see for yourself. Nothing like a processed meal that can likely sit on your shelf for a year, maybe two. Think about that.

Converting calories to another system of measurement is still tracking calories, it's simply less transparent because you're not aware of the caloric intake once you're done with that plan. And telling people not to bother counting calories at all, as some programs do, is a terrible practice. These tactics are born to keep you on the hook, not to help you manage your weight moving forward. And knowing some basic caloric values isn't as hard as many diet plans would like you to believe.

The Cucumber Diet specifies calories for every recipe so you can begin to gain awareness about the caloric cost of what you eat. Once you do, calorie management becomes innate.

Think about it this way. Would you go shopping without having a budget or buy groceries without knowing the prices? Of course not. Math is our friend, and it's a tool we use every day. If you buy milk, you have an idea of what milk costs. It may vary a bit, but it's reasonably consistent.

It works the same way with food. A hard-boiled egg is about 78 calories. A two-egg omelet is about 160 calories. Include a few reasonable add-ins, and it's about 225-250 calories. Most of us have favorites, so it's easy to get to know a handful of caloric values once you've practiced conscious eating for a little while.

Managing Calories

Personally, I like to manage calories by the day. If I want to shift calories around from lunch to dinner, for example, I can, but it's not a hard and fast rule. What matters most at the end of the day is that I know what my total daily caloric intake is. The important thing to remember is that nothing, water aside, is calorie-free. Everything counts. Once you know that, you can make more informed decisions about what and how much you eat.

Of course, it's important to note that like foods, not all calories are created equal. Whole foods and low-calorie-density foods are generally a better value than junk food or highly processed snacks.

The daily calories allocated in our plan are based on the U.S average number of calories. The actual number of calories that's right for you depends on a few factors including age, weight, height, your activity level, and general metabolic health. I suggest going online and searching "Mifflin-St. JEOR equation". The Mifflin-St. JEOR equation is a very basic calculator available online.[18] You'll answer a few questions, and it will give you a precise number of calories you need a day to maintain or lose weight.

For example, I am on the smaller side of an active, average male. The national average would put me at 2500 calories to maintain, and 2000 to lose weight. But the Mifflin-St. JEOR equation calculator puts me at 2153 calories to maintain, and 1722 to lose. If I consumed an average of 2500 calories a day, I would be gaining weight. Over time, I found the right number for me is around 2000 calories a day, closer to where the Mifflin-St. JEOR equation put me.

At roughly 2000 calories a day I maintain my weight, but also I give myself a five-pound variance. If I gain close to 5 pounds, I knock the calories back to 1700 until I pull myself back into my comfort zone. I find that being able to maintain my weight easily is empowering. Once you have good habits established, conscious eating comes naturally.

The Cucumber Diet is based on 1500 calories a day for women and 1900 calories a day for men. So determine the right number of daily calories for you. If your daily caloric needs vary from the national average, you may need more or less calories than our daily allocation. If so, modify your daily allocations slightly up or down accordingly.

Whatever you do, don't get crazy about one day's worth of calories, just as long as a week balances out. For example, if I have a 2500 or 2800 calorie day, the next day or two I will consume fewer calories. On a weekly basis, I strive to average 2000 calories a day. It's essential that you don't punish yourself for weak moments or worse yet, give up on your goals entirely. You can do this.

How many calories are in the Cucumber Diet?

We've done the math and designed the Cucumber Diet to meet a caloric allocation that is targeted for weight loss. Because we've made the caloric management of the plan transparent, it will give you a chance to establish better habits and maintain your weight loss long term.

The Cucumber Diet is based on 1500 calories for women and 1900 calories a day for men to lose weight, divided among meals into the following average range.

Women

Breakfast: (250 calories)

Lunch: (450 calories)

Dinner: (150) + (500) (650 calories)

Dessert: (150 calories)

Men

Breakfast: (250 calories)

Lunch: (600 calories)

Dinner: (150) + (750) (900 calories)

Dessert: (150 calories)

You can use this basic meal allocation for the Cucumber Diet and modify to your caloric preferences. Doing the math is an exercise in gaining awareness of calories. You won't always have to count the caloric cost, but If you follow this plan for a few months, you can begin to assess and allocate calories until it comes naturally.

Once you've reached your goal, maintaining your weight on the Cucumber Diet is easy. You can gradually add some flexibility to your daily menu, adapting your allocations based on the calories you need to maintain weight. Continue to focus on serving size but don't stress about the extra bite or two of dessert. We'll talk more about additional ways to maintain your weight loss by introducing some exercise into your daily routine later in the book.

While the Cucumber Diet does not make any specific weight loss claims, it is a calorie restricted plan. With respect to calories and weight loss, it is widely accepted that the following rule of 3,500 calories is about one pound. According to the Mayo Clinic:

"Because 3,500 calories equals about 1 pound (0.45 kilogram) of fat, it's estimated that you need to burn about 3,500 calories to lose 1 pound. So, in general, if you cut about 500 to 1,000 calories a day from your typical diet, you'd lose about 1 to 2 pounds a week."[19]

11 Griffin, R. Morgan. "Healthy Whole Foods: Making Nutrient-Rich Choices for Your Diet." WebMD, WebMD, https://www.webmd.com/diet/features/the-benefits-of-healthy-whole-foods#1

12 Stanhope, Kimber L, et al. "Adverse Metabolic Effects of Dietary Fructose: Results from the Recent Epidemiological, Clinical, and Mechanistic Studies." Current Opinion in Lipidology, U.S. National Library of Medicine, June 2013, www.ncbi.nlm.nih.gov/pubmed/23594708

13 Wanders, A J, et al. "Effects of Dietary Fibre on Subjective Appetite, Energy Intake and Body Weight: a Systematic Review of Randomized Controlled Trials." Obesity Reviews : an Official Journal of the International Association for the Study of Obesity, U.S. National Library of Medicine, Sept. 2011, www.ncbi.nlm.nih.gov/pubmed/21676152

14 Romaguera, Dora, et al. "Dietary Determinants of Changes in Waist Circumference Adjusted for Body Mass Index - a Proxy Measure of Visceral Adiposity." PloS One, Public Library of Science, 14 July 2010, https://www.ncbi.nlm.nih.gov/pubmed/20644647

15 Ello-Martin, Julia A, et al. "Dietary Energy Density in the Treatment of Obesity: a Year-Long Trial Comparing 2 Weight-Loss Diets." The American Journal of Clinical Nutrition, U.S. National Library of Medicine, June 2007, https://www.ncbi.nlm.nih.gov/pmc/articles/PMC2018610

16 Klatell, Penny. "How Big Are Your Dinner Plates - And Why It Matters." Eat Out Eat Well, 15 Oct. 2012, https://eatouteatwell.com/how-big-are-your-dinner-plates-and-why-it-matters/

17 Khazan, Olga. "We Eat 92 Percent of the Food on Our Plates." The Atlantic, Atlantic Media Company, 25 July 2014, https://www.theatlantic.com/health/archive/2014/07/we-eat-92-percent-of-the-food-on-our-plates/375016/

18 Frankenfield, David C. "Bias and Accuracy of Resting Metabolic Rate Equations in Non-Obese and Obese Adults." Clinical Nutrition Journal, Dec. 2013, https://www.clinicalnutritionjournal.com/article/S0261-5614(13)00100-3/abstract

19 "The Best Ways to Cut Calories from Your Diet." Mayo Clinic, Mayo Foundation for Medical Education and Research, 28 Mar. 2018, https://www.mayoclinic.org/healthy-lifestyle/weight-loss/in-depth/calories/art-20048065

The Cucumber Diet Plan

Having a weight loss strategy that is rooted in science is critical, but you also need a plan so you can implement best practices like consuming low-calorie-density foods to reach your goals. That's where the Cucumber Diet comes in. It's a simple, straightforward diet with flexible, easy to prepare meals that will help you stay within an optimal caloric range that promotes weight loss. For women, that caloric range is about 1500 calories. For men, it's about 1900 calories.

The Cucumber Diet consists of three meals plus dessert. Yep. You heard that right. Dessert is still on the menu. Because this isn't just a diet, it's a lifestyle. And learning how to have the sweet stuff in moderation is essential for not only losing weight but keeping it off.

It's the same for alcohol: if you enjoy a drink you can still have it!

Keep in mind sugary alcoholic drinks, the kind with the little umbrellas you see poolside can have an entire meal's worth of calories in one glass. If a high calorie drink can be an entire meal, drinking a few certainly suggests you could be drinking your calories and then some. It is very, very easy to drink your calories. Measure and add club soda or extra ice to extend and drink less alcohol.

To avoid this calorie trap, consider ordering your next cocktail as a "reverse pour." The reverse pour strategy involves ordering your martini or cosmopolitan as you normally would and asking for a large glass of ice on the side. Instead of putting the ice in your drink, pour your drink over the ice. Half of your drink will probably fill the glass, effectively stretching one drink into two.

Once you begin the cucumber diet, do your best not to stray too far off plan into substitutions, at least at first. Because you're retraining yourself in the art of conscious eating, it will take some time for your palate, and your serving sizes to catch up. In the interim, following the plan will help you to establish healthy habits and put you on the road to the lifestyle you crave.

Life is busy, and you don't always have the time or the ingredients to whip up a full meal in the comfort of your own kitchen. That's why each recipe section also identifies quick, grab-n-go solutions that you can purchase without wandering off-plan. Whether you're eating breakfast in the car because you're running late or trying to cram dinner in before helping the kids with their homework, you won't have to sacrifice your well-being for convenience.

About Ingredients

You will see in our recipes that many use only ingredients that are very familiar to everyone, ingredients you likely already have or that are easy to find in any grocery store. Some ingredients are less common and may even be unfamiliar to you: whey, almond milk, chia seeds or Greek yogurt. You can find these ingredients in most local supermarkets and we encourage you to try some of them: new foods and new recipes will make the diet more adventurous and interesting as you change your eating habits and cultivate conscious eating. Fresh vegetables make all the difference. Find a store that has good produce and make a habit of shopping there. The difference will be worth it. And remember, our goal is conscious eating: it is good to think about your food. Not in a guilty or worried way, but by being interested and enjoying what you eat.

Breakfast: Rise and Shine

They say breakfast is the most important meal of the day and who are we to argue. The Cucumber Diet breakfast recipes have something for everyone, with an emphasis on well-rounded meals that include whole grains, fruits, and small amounts of healthy fat to keep you satisfied until lunch.

You'll discover most of our breakfast recipes fall within the 250 caloric range, with ingredients you can find in any supermarket. On average, these meals take about 10 minutes to prepare, but you can certainly make some items, such as chia pudding or pancakes, the night before. And as always, if you're pressed for time, you can find our list of quick, grab-n-go solutions at the end of this section.

Almond Butter Is My Jam Smoothie

Got a hankering for peanut butter and jelly? Get your fix with this smooth spin on a lunch box favorite. **Calories: 272**

½ cup frozen strawberries

½ cup frozen raspberries

¼ cup original, unsweetened almond milk

1 Tbsp. almond butter

1 Tbsp. quick oats oatmeal, uncooked

Pinch of kosher salt

Directions: *Put ingredients in a blender. Blend until smooth and enjoy immediately.*

A word about nut butters…If you don't have almond butter on hand, it's okay to use peanut butter, cashew butter, or even walnut butter as a substitution. But be aware that different nuts and nut butters have different health properties to keep in mind.

- Walnut butter has the least calories per serving, sliding in at just 85 calories per tablespoon.
- Need protein? Stick with peanut or almond butter because they boast 7 grams of protein per serving.
- If you're looking for the least fat, walnut butter is just 14 grams per serving with the highest levels of Omega-3 (yes, those are the good fats).
- When it comes to vitamin content, almond butter packs a punch with more than 52% of your daily value of Vitamin E in just two tablespoons.
- Cashew butter gives a boost to mineral levels with higher levels of both magnesium and copper than other nut butters.[20]

Now that you're better informed, you can pick a nut butter that'll give you the most bang for your calorie buck.

20 Martinac, Paula. "What Is the Healthiest Nut Butter?" Healthy Eating | SF Gate, 6 Dec. 2018, https://healthyeating.sfgate.com/healthiest-nut-butter-10096.html.

Basil Blueberry Smoothie

This quickie breakfast in a glass features the amazing combination of blueberries and basil and an extra punch of protein to keep you going until lunch. **Calories: 274 calories**

1 cup frozen blueberries

1/4 cup loosely packed basil leaves

1/3 cup original, unsweetened almond milk

2 Tbsp. Greek yogurt

½ Tbsp. honey

1 scoop of vanilla or plain whey protein powder

¼ - ½ cup cold water until desired consistency

Directions: *Put all ingredients except water into a blender. Blend until smooth, gradually adding water as needed to reach desired consistency. Enjoy immediately.*

Smoothie Substitutions: Don't have an ingredient in your pantry or fridge? No problem. Smoothies are adaptable. You can use any kind of berry, switch out a different herb, and mix in any kind of milk that floats your boat. Just watch your calorie count to make sure you keep as close as possible to that sweet spot of 250-300 calories.

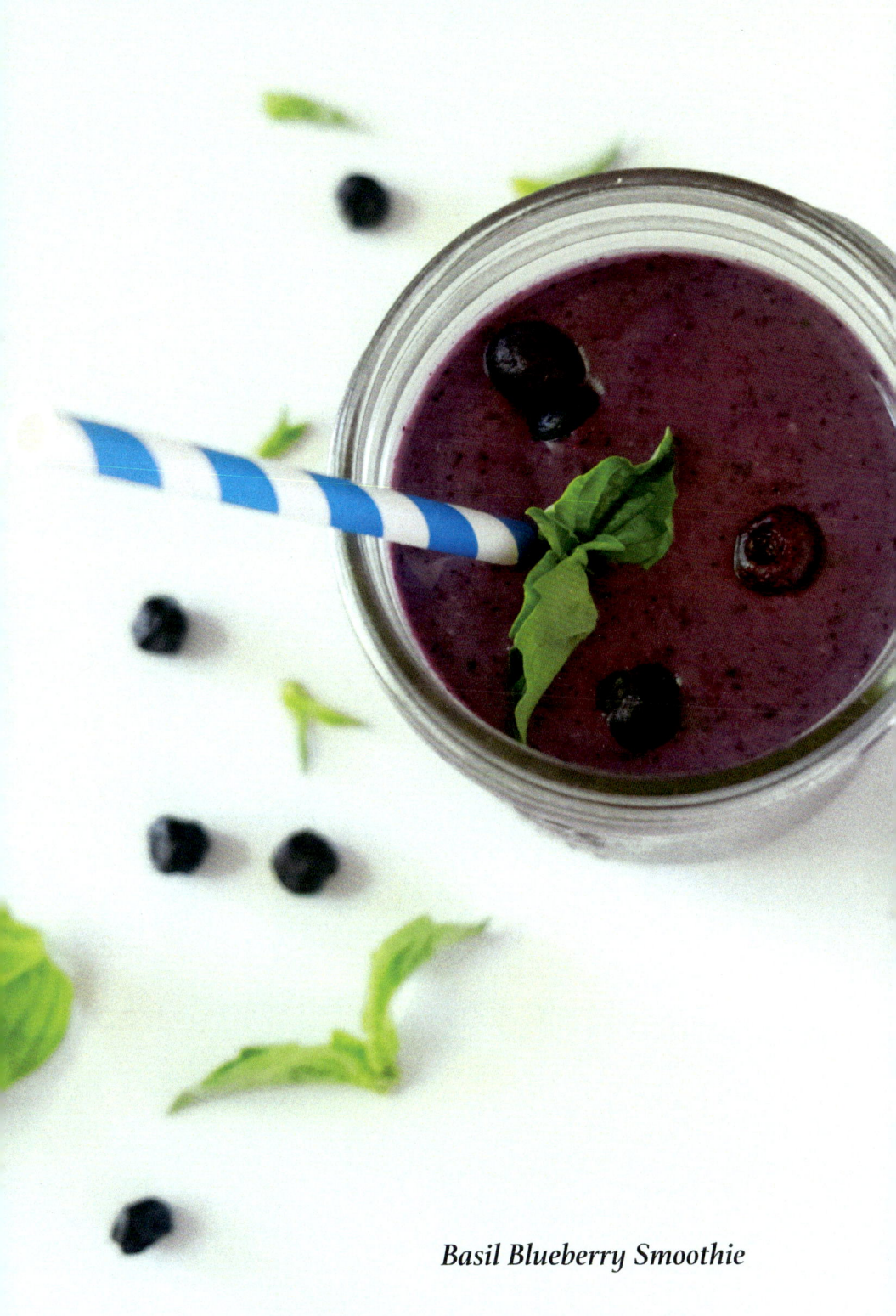

Basil Blueberry Smoothie

9-Minute Shakshuka

This version of shakshuka is a breeze to whip up. Use fresh tomatoes when possible, but canned will do in a pinch. **Calories: 245**

½ **Tbsp extra-virgin olive oil**

¼ **cup sliced green onions**

½ **tsp. minced garlic**

¼ **tsp. ground cumin**

1/3 **cup chopped tomatoes**

2 **cups fresh spinach**

2 **Tbsp. water**

2 **eggs**

1 **Tbsp. feta cheese**

Pinch of salt

¼ **cup chopped parsley, mint or cilantro for garnish**

Directions: *Heat oil in a skillet over medium heat. Add green onions, garlic, and cumin, stirring and cooking until fragrant about 30 seconds. Add tomatoes and stir until they break down about 3 minutes. Add spinach and water and stir for about 30 seconds until wilted. Add salt. Crack two eggs over vegetables, cover and let steam over medium-low until eggs are set about three minutes. Remove from stove, sprinkle with feta and let stand for 2 minutes before serving. Garnish with mint, parsley, or cilantro.*

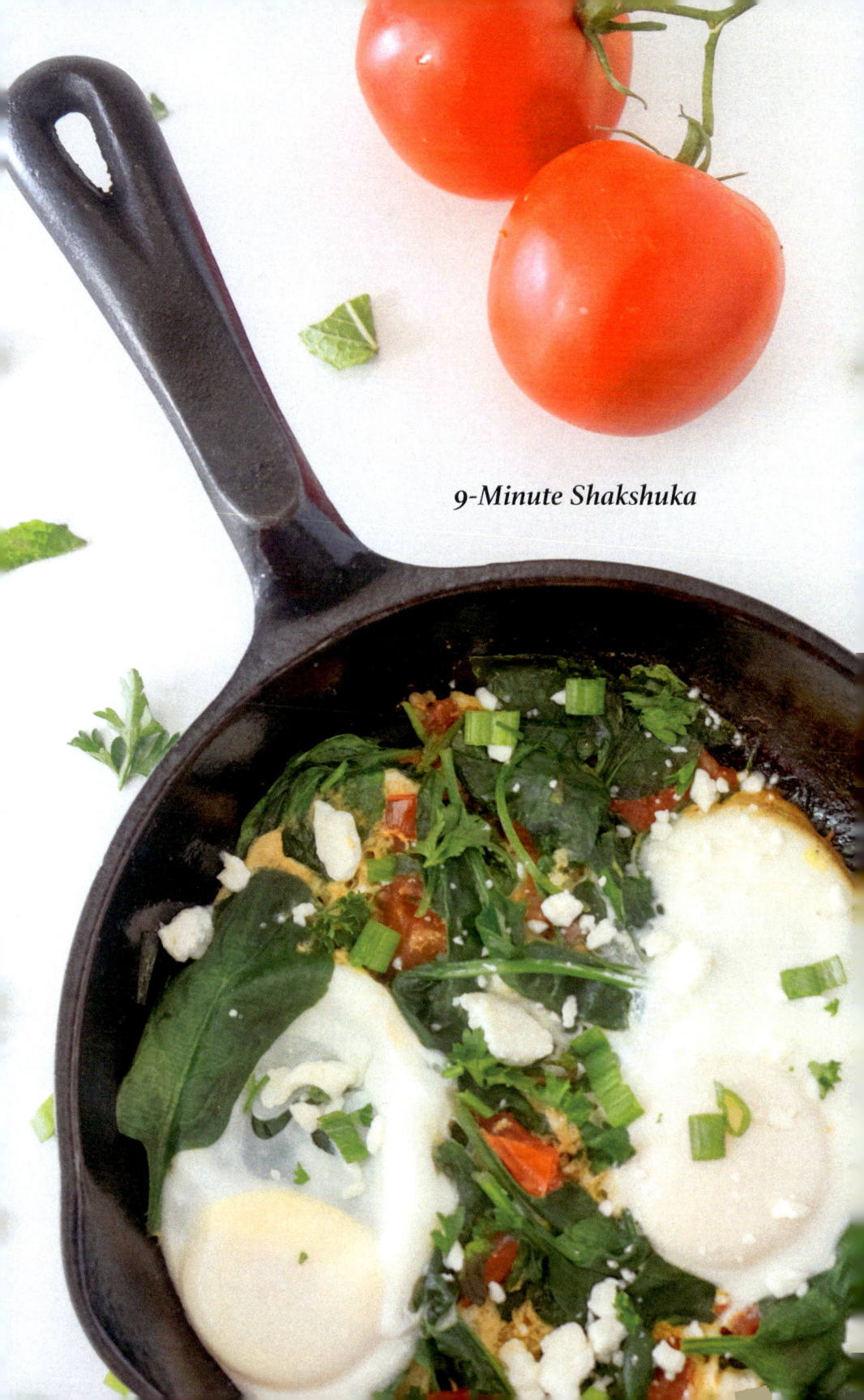

9-Minute Shakshuka

Eggs & Things

Quickie Eggs in a Mug

For a healthy, savory bite of eggs try this quick microwave version that's a convenient alternative to an omelet. **Calories: 250**

2 eggs

2 Tbsp sundried tomatoes

¼ cup diced ham

¼ cup spinach

2 Tbsp. feta cheese

1 tsp. sliced green onions

Cooking spray

Salt & pepper to taste

Directions: *Spray inside of a mug with cooking spray. Crack eggs into mug, using a fork to whip the yolks and whites together. Add sundried tomatoes, spinach, feta, ham and green onions as well as salt and pepper. Stir. Microwave mug on high for one minute and 30 seconds. Remove and let sit for one minute before eating.*

French Herbed Eggs with Cream

It sounds decadent, but the secret to enjoying these baked eggs is moderation. **Calories: 250**

¼ tsp minced garlic

¼ tsp. thyme or rosemary

½ Tbsp. fresh parsley

½ Tbsp parmesan cheese

2 eggs

½ Tbsp. heavy cream

½ Tbsp. unsalted butter

Salt & pepper to taste

Directions: *Preheat broiler and place rack 6 inches from heat. Combine garlic, herbs, and parmesan in a small bowl. Put a ramekin or oven-safe bowl on a baking sheet. Place cream and butter in the dish, then place under the broiler for 2-3 minutes until it bubbles. Crack eggs into ramekin and sprinkle with herb and cheese mixture. Salt and pepper to taste. Put back under broiler for 4-5 minutes, then remove from heat as soon as whites are set. Cool before eating.*

The Big Greek Egg Sandwich

A hearty breakfast begins with a healthy dose of eggs and flavorful mix-ins like roasted red peppers and feta on an open-faced sandwich.
Calories: 298

½ Tbsp. olive oil

½ tsp. minced garlic

1/3 cup roasted red peppers, chopped

2 eggs

1 Tbsp. feta cheese

1 slice whole-wheat bread

Fresh, chopped parsley

Salt & pepper to taste

Directions: *In a skillet over medium heat, warm olive oil. Add garlic and peppers and cook one minute until fragrant. Crack eggs into the skillet and sprinkle with feta and salt & pepper. Cover and cook until eggs are set, about 5-8 minutes. Top piece of toasted wheat bread with eggs and sprinkle with parsley.*

Blue Cheese & Bacon Egg Muffins

Indulge in a little extra with these easy to make egg muffins, crammed with blue cheese, bacon, and spinach. **Calories: 247**

2 eggs

¼ cup fresh spinach

1 Tbsp. crumbled bacon

¼ cup crumbled blue cheese

Cooking spray

Salt & pepper to taste

Directions: *Preheat oven to 350 degrees. While it's warming, coat muffin tin with cooking spray. Whisk eggs with spinach, bacon, and cheese. Divide between two muffin cups. Bake 12-15 minutes until set. Cool before eating.*

Garden Quinoa Cups

Make a big batch of these quinoa cups and nibble them all week long for a healthy, savory breakfast packed with good stuff from the garden. **Calories: 292, serving size 2 cups**

2 cups cooked quinoa

2 eggs

2 egg whites

1 cup shredded zucchini

1/2 cup shredded cheddar cheese

1/3 cup diced turkey

¼ cup chopped parsley

¼ cup green onions, chopped

Salt & pepper to taste

Cooking spray

Directions: Heat oven to 375 degrees. Coat a muffin tin with cooking spray. Combine quinoa, eggs, egg whites, zucchini, cheddar cheese, turkey, parsley, and green onions in a large bowl. Whisk together. Season with salt and pepper, then pour evenly into 12 muffin cups. Bake 12-25 minutes. Makes 6 servings.

Cashew Apple Oatmeal Snack Cups

These little cups pack a big wallop of nutrition with applesauce and oatmeal and the extra nutty flavor of cashew butter. **Calories: 243, serving size 3 cups**

1/2 cup applesauce

2 eggs

1 tsp. vanilla extract

1/2 cup unsweetened almond milk

2 cups quick-cook oats, uncooked

1 tsp. baking powder

2 Tbsp. coconut oil

2 tbsp. cashew butter

Cooking spray

Directions: Preheat oven to 350 degrees and spray a muffin tin with cooking spray. Stir together applesauce, eggs, vanilla extract, and almond milk. Whisk until well combined. Add the oatmeal, baking powder, and coconut oil, and mix until smooth. Fill muffin tins about 1/3 to 1/2 way full. Sprinkle with additional oats for texture on top. Bake at 350 for about 18-20 minutes. Top with a dollop of cashew butter when serving. Makes 12 snack cups.

Peach-Puffed Oven Pancake

Think you have to give up pancakes? Think again. This healthy pancake recipe features fresh peaches with a touch of butter and brown sugar. **Calories: 250, serving size 2 wedges**

1 Tbsp. butter

3 eggs

½ cup all-purpose flour

½ cup skim milk

¼ tsp. cinnamon

Pinch of salt

2 medium peaches, thinly sliced

2 Tbsp. brown sugar

2 tsp. water

Cooking spray

Directions: *Heat oven to 400 degrees. Place butter in oven-safe skillet until it melts and bubbles. Whisk eggs, flour, milk, cinnamon, and salt in a large bowl until smooth. Pour batter into skillet. Bake 20-25 minutes until browned.*

Coat saucepan with cooking spray and warm on medium heat. Add peaches, brown sugar, and water. Cook 4-6 minutes until peaches begin to break down, stirring occasionally. Spoon peach mixture over pancake. Cut into 8 wedges.

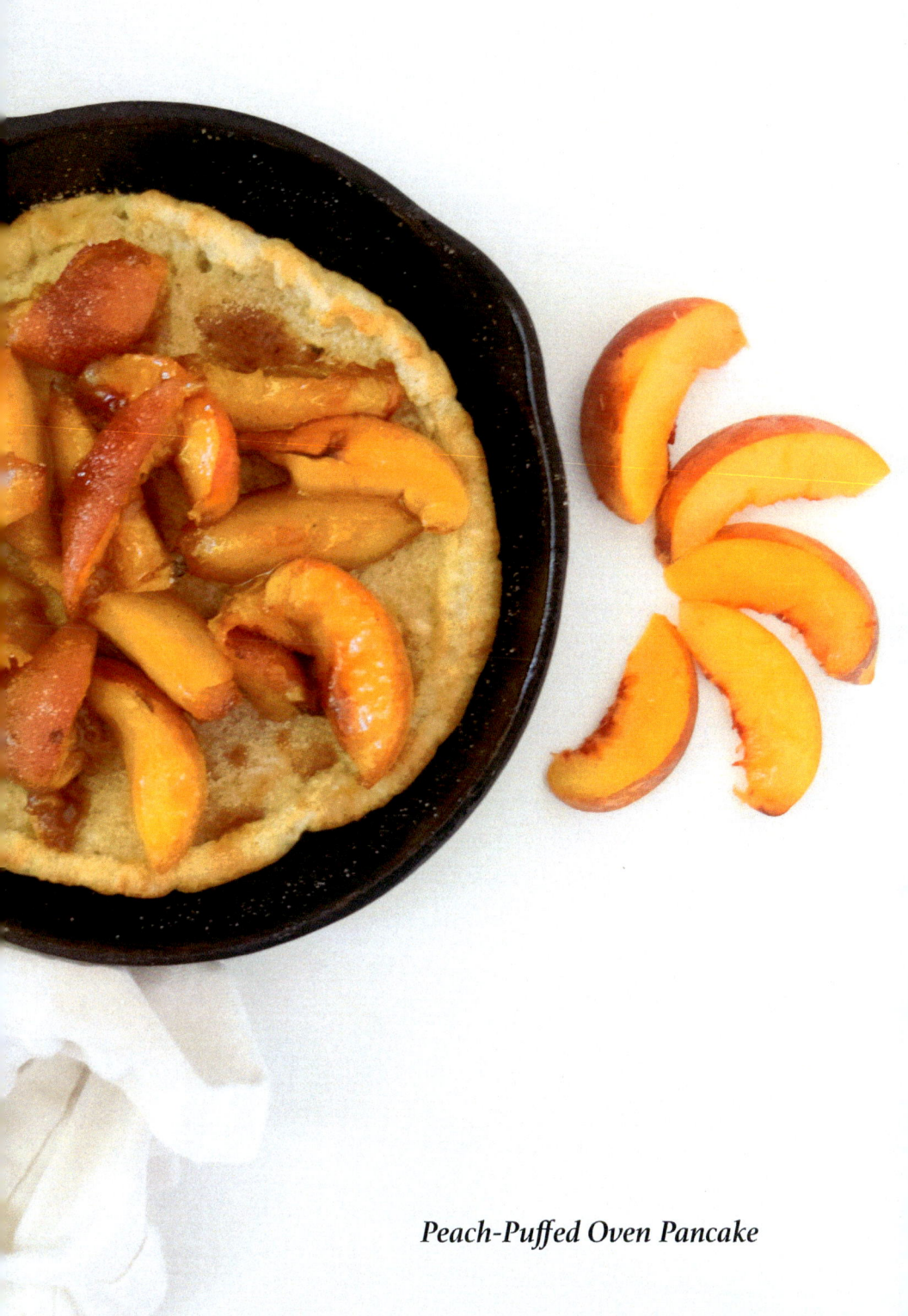

Peach-Puffed Oven Pancake

Chocolate Coconut Chia Pudding

Chocolate for breakfast? Don't mind if I do. This perfect pairing of chocolate and coconut lets chia seeds show off as the delectable nuggets of nutrients they are. **Calories: 264**

¼ cup cocoa powder

1 Tbsp. maple syrup

½ tsp ground cardamom

Pinch of salt

¼ tsp. vanilla extract

3/4 cup unsweetened coconut milk

1/3 cup chia seeds

Pinch of shaved coconut

Directions: In a bowl, toss cocoa, cardamom and salt then mix in maple syrup and vanilla. Add coconut milk slowly, forming a paste and then continuing to whisk until smooth. Add chia seeds. Cover and refrigerate overnight or at least 3-5 hours until the pudding is set. Keeps 4-5 days but best when served fresh. Sprinkle with a pinch of shaved coconut

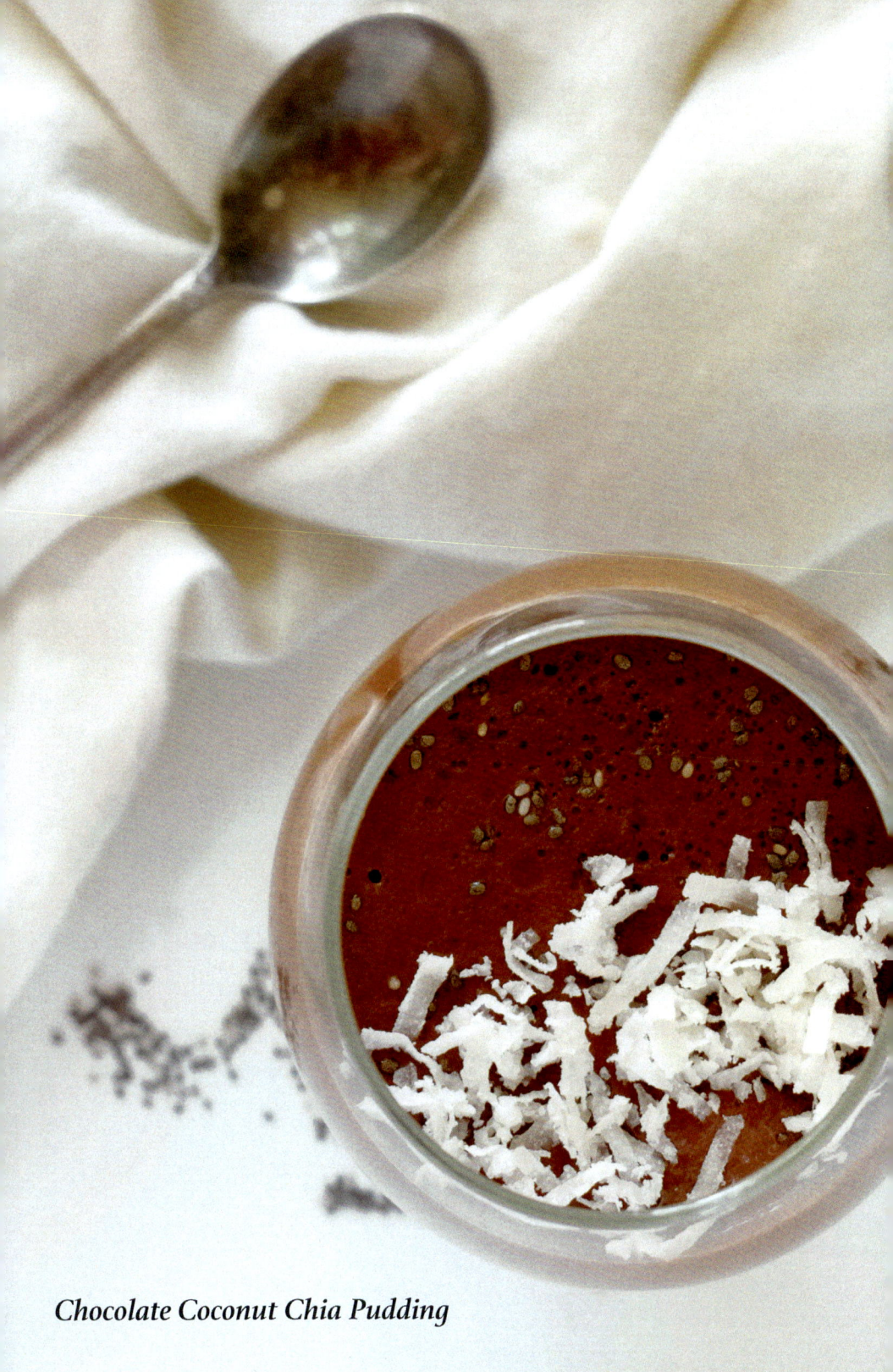

Chocolate Coconut Chia Pudding

Chia & Cashew Butter Toast

A quick solution for a hectic morning, chia toast is always ready to satisfy at a moment's notice. **Calories: 232**

1 Tbsp. cashew butter

1 slice whole-wheat bread, toasted

½ tsp. chia seeds

Pinch of cinnamon

Directions: *Spread cashew butter over bread, then sprinkle with chia seeds and cinnamon.*

Sunny-Side Up Avocado Toast

This breakfast loaded with healthy fats and whole grains is always ready to help you greet the day. **Calories: 243**

1 slice whole-wheat bread

¼ small avocado, mashed

1 large egg

Salt & pepper to taste

Microgreens

Cooking spray

Directions: *Mash avocado and season to taste with salt and pepper. Coat a small skillet with cooking spray and heat on low. Crack an egg into skillet, cover, and cook until set. Toast whole-wheat bread, then top with avocado, egg, and microgreens.*

Banana Almond Butter Chia Seed Pudding

If you've got some ripe bananas and a little almond butter, we've got a great idea. **Calories: 302**

1 ripe banana

1/2 cup almond milk

½ Tbsp almond butter

1 Tbsp. chia seeds

Directions: *In a blender, puree banana, almond milk, and almond butter. Transfer to a bowl and stir in chia seeds. Cover with plastic wrap and chill overnight or for at least 4 hours. Can be stored up to one week.*

Why chia seeds? Chia seeds are all the rage for a reason. These wee things pack a wallop both in terms of fiber and Omega-3s. Just a one ounce serving of this superfood provides the following:

- 11 grams of fiber
- 4 grams of protein
- 9 grams of fat, 5 of which are Omega-3 heart-healthy fats
- 18% of your daily value of calcium
- 30% of your daily value of magnesium

Not to mention plenty of other nutrients such as phosphorus, manganese, zinc, and potassium. Loaded with antioxidants, chia seeds are one of the world's best sources per calorie for several essential vitamins and minerals. So don't be shy about sprinkling those chia seeds around.[21]

21 Megan Ware, RDN. "Chia Seeds: Health Benefits and Recipe Tips." Medical News Today, MediLexicon International, 12 Nov. 2018, https://www.medicalnewstoday.com/articles/291334.php

Plum & Almond Baked Oatmeal

This oatmeal for a crowd is packed with plums and can be prepared ahead of time for a quick reheat. **Calories: 349**

2 cups rolled oats, uncooked

1/4 cup light brown sugar

1/2 teaspoon salt

1 teaspoon baking powder

1 teaspoon ground cinnamon

1/3 cup chopped almonds

2 cups Unsweetened Almond Milk

1 large egg

2 tablespoons coconut oil melted and cooled slightly (or melted and cooled butter)

1 teaspoon almond extract

1 1/2 cups chopped plums

Cooking spray

Directions: *Preheat the oven to 350 degrees. Spray an 8x8 square baking dish with cooking spray and set aside. In a medium bowl, mix the oats, brown sugar, baking powder, salt, cinnamon, and almonds. In another bowl, whisk the almond milk, egg, coconut oil, and almond extract.*

Arrange the chopped plums on the bottom of the prepared baking dish. Pour the oat mixture evenly over the plums. Pour the almond milk mixture over the oats. Gently shake the baking dish to make sure the milk covers the oats evenly. Bake for 40 minutes, until the top is golden and oatmeal is set. Let cool for 5 minutes and serve warm.

Grab-n-Go Breakfasts

Sometimes, your morning doesn't go according to plan. Stay on track by purchasing some of these off-the-shelf supermarket solutions that fall between 200-250 calories.

Make your own yogurt parfait

Purchase a small, single-serving size container of low-fat Greek yogurt and a small box or pouch of high fiber cereal, such as All-Bran Buds, Fiber One, All-Bran or Grape-Nuts. About ¼ cup of cereal added to the top of your yogurt container makes a fine breakfast on the run.

Add a little fruit to the mix

If you want to stay on the sweet side of your calorie count, opt for fruit as a mix-in for your yogurt instead of cereal or granola. Many fruits like berries are low-calorie-density foods, and you can afford to eat a healthy handful or two with your yogurt and not worry about your waistline.

Channel your childhood with cereal

When in doubt, fill your bowl with a standby like cereal. Instead of choosing colorful, sugary solutions stick with a single serving size of granolas and high fiber cereals. While they may be higher in calorie count, these smaller portion cereals have lots more substance and will keep you fuller longer. Opt for almond, coconut, or regular milk but take it easy on the pour.

Go wholesome with oatmeal

Oatmeal gets a bad rap as a boring breakfast food, but it's likely you've just been eating it wrong. Swing by a Starbucks and try their classic oatmeal to give you a new appreciate of how dried fruit and a little sugar can transform steel cut oats into a satisfying, warm breakfast in a cup.

Cucumber Bowl Lunch:

Fill Your Bowl with The Good Stuff

You need fuel to face your busy day, so we've designed lunch to deliver. The centerpiece of this diet is our flavorful, satisfying cucumber bowls overflowing with low-calorie dense foods. They're fast and simple to make, flexible, and built on a broad range of ingredients that you can customize to suit your taste buds.

Our carefully crafted Cucumber Bowl recipes provide exciting flavor combinations, from Baja to Morocco. In addition to the recipes provided, the handy chart will help you mix and match to build your own cucumber bowl so you can discover new favorites.

While several dressing recipes are included, you're also free to purchase dressings in a bottle to make your prep a little easier. On average, even with the chopping and dicing, it'll take about ten minutes to assemble your cucumber bowl.

A word about prep

There are two things you can do to make preparing cucumber bowls quick and convenient, whether you're eating at home or hauling them to work. First, print out the chart and bring it with you shopping. Stock up on non-perishables like quinoa, lentils, rice, oils, and dressings, so you'll have what you need to assemble a bowl on hand.

Secondly, making a little time to prepare for the week is definitely the way to go. Plan out your daily bowls and slice, dice, and chop your items ahead of time. For instance, keeping a supply of hard-boiled eggs, sliced olives, and cooked quinoa and rice on hand will really cut down on prep time and allow you to incorporate variety into your meals.

You should also feel inspired to spice it up as you prepare your cucumber bowl ingredients. Using a little taco seasoning or cumin to season your cooked chicken breast or garnishing your finished bowl with herbs, microgreens, or a squeeze of lime or lemon juice is always welcome. These kinds of variations are listed under freebies, and they'll make you feel like you're indulging.

When it comes to meat like chicken and other items that fall under Category B from the chart, cooking ahead storing in the fridge is optimal. If that's not practical, Applegate brand is a good go-to for organic, sliced meats without antibiotics that are minimally processed. For the Cucumber Diet, three slices of Applegate meats are usually a serving size but check the package to be sure you're staying within the same caloric range as indicated on the chart.

As you prepare your bowl, you should also pay attention to the most critical ingredient. Your cucumbers should be fresh and retain some skin to deliver maximum nutrients and flavor. You can peel a little from the skin in strips if you've got a particularly tough one on hand but otherwise strive to keep some skin in the game to get the most out of your lunchtime calories.

Beware the dressing dilemma

One of the easiest ways to overdo it is to go overboard on the dressing. It happens to everyone. Cucumbers are refreshing and crisp, and their flavors play well with others, so a bit of balsamic vinegar and olive oil offer a lot of bang for your buck. If you want a quick alternative from the grocery store shelf, organic dressings labeled "light" are your best bet.

One serving of dressing is two tablespoons, and in the beginning, you shouldn't trust yourself to eyeball it. Measure it until you get the hang of what a serving size is. After you've adjusted, you can go back to pouring it out of the bottle with this little trick. Every time you pour a serving of dressing put a small notch on the label or bottle with a marker. If a bottle is 16 servings and you don't have 16 notches, you've been like your favorite bartender. A little too generous with the pour.

Cucumber Bowl Recipes

Take the guesswork out of lunch with our handy build-your-own chart at the end of the lunch section. Mix and match three veggies, two protein sources, and a bit of fat with your cucumber. Then top with dressing and throw in a few freebies for flavor. You'll be surprised at how delicious and filling those extra mouthfuls can be.

The Baja Cucumber Bowl

A Mexican inspired cucumber bowl will add a little spice to your lunch hour with all the fixings of your favorite burrito. **382 calories**

1 hydroponic cucumber, sliced

1/2 onion, diced

1 tomato chopped

1 bell pepper, diced

½ cooked chicken breast, sliced or chopped

½ cup black beans

2 Tbsp. cheddar cheese

Cilantro lime dressing:

¼ cup chopped cilantro

½ Tbsp. avocado oil

1-2 tsp. lime juice

1 Tbsp. white vinegar

1-2 dashes hot sauce (optional)

Directions: Assemble your chopped and diced veggies in a bowl. Arrange chicken breast on top, sprinkle with black beans and cheese. Drizzle with cilantro lime dressing. Sprinkle with cilantro if desired.

For the cilantro lime dressing: In a food processor, pulse cilantro, avocado oil, lime juice, vinegar, and hot sauce to taste until smooth. Keep refrigerated.

Alternate bottled dressing: Fat-free Catalina

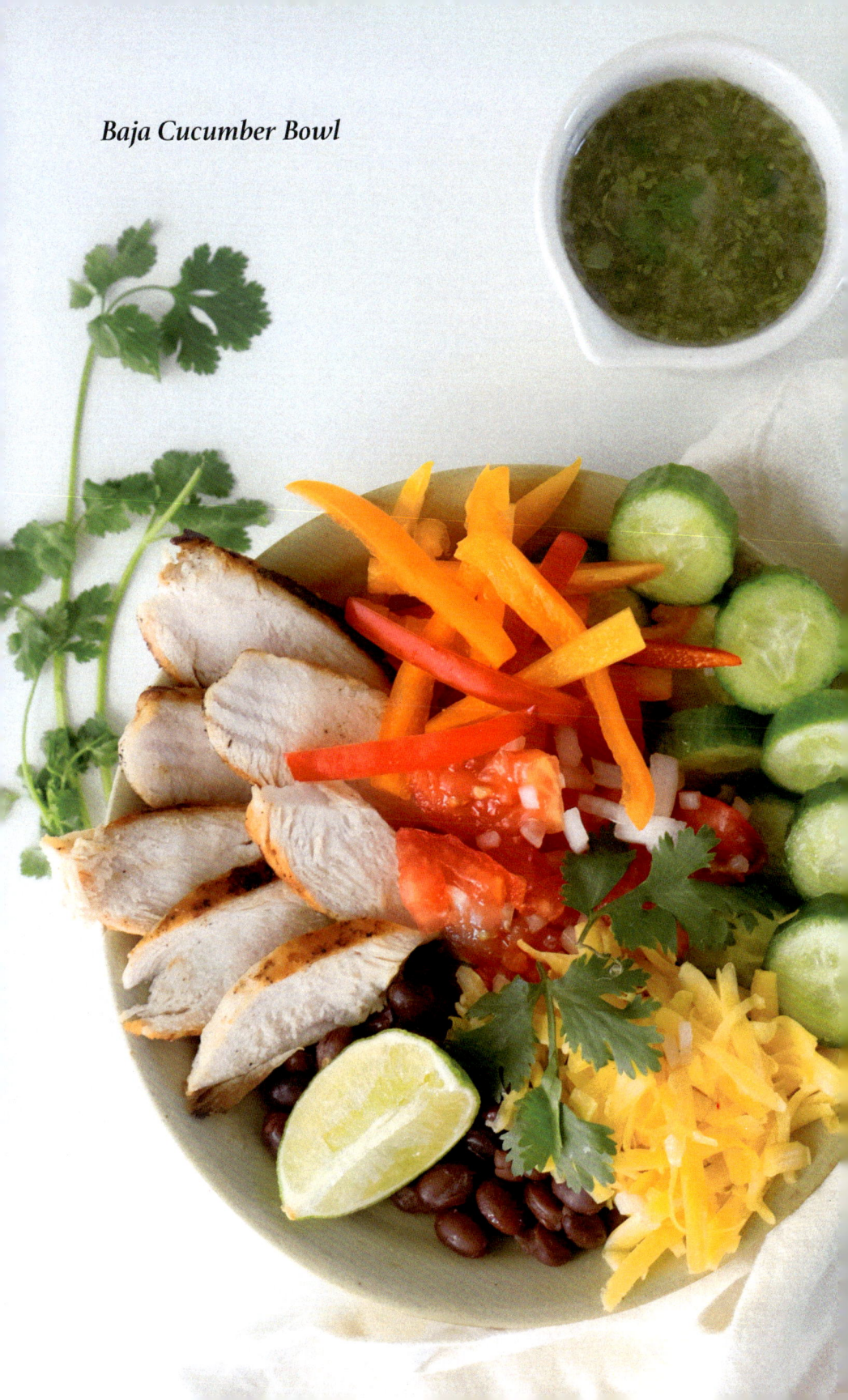

Baja Cucumber Bowl

The Niçoise Cucumber Bowl

This cucumber bowl is a spin on a French classic, featuring a cucumber base, olives, microgreens, and a lemon mustard dressing. **353 calories**

1 hydroponic cucumber, sliced

1 tomato, chopped

1 can (4 oz.) of tuna in water, drained

1 hard-boiled egg, sliced

¼ cup sliced black olives

Lemon mustard dressing:

2 Tbsp. lemon juice

1 tsp. mustard

½ tsp extra-virgin olive oil

1 Tbsp. white wine vinegar

Salt & pepper

Microgreens

Directions: Put sliced cucumbers in a bowl. Prepare your chopped tomatoes and toss on top. Arrange drained tuna and hard-boiled egg slices in a bowl, then sprinkle with black olives. Drizzle with lemon mustard dressing and garnish with microgreens if desired.

For the lemon mustard dressing: Put lemon juice, mustard, extra-virgin olive oil, vinegar, and salt and pepper in a mason jar with a lid. Fasten the lid securely and shake until combined well. Keep refrigerated.

Alternate bottled dressing: Light Italian

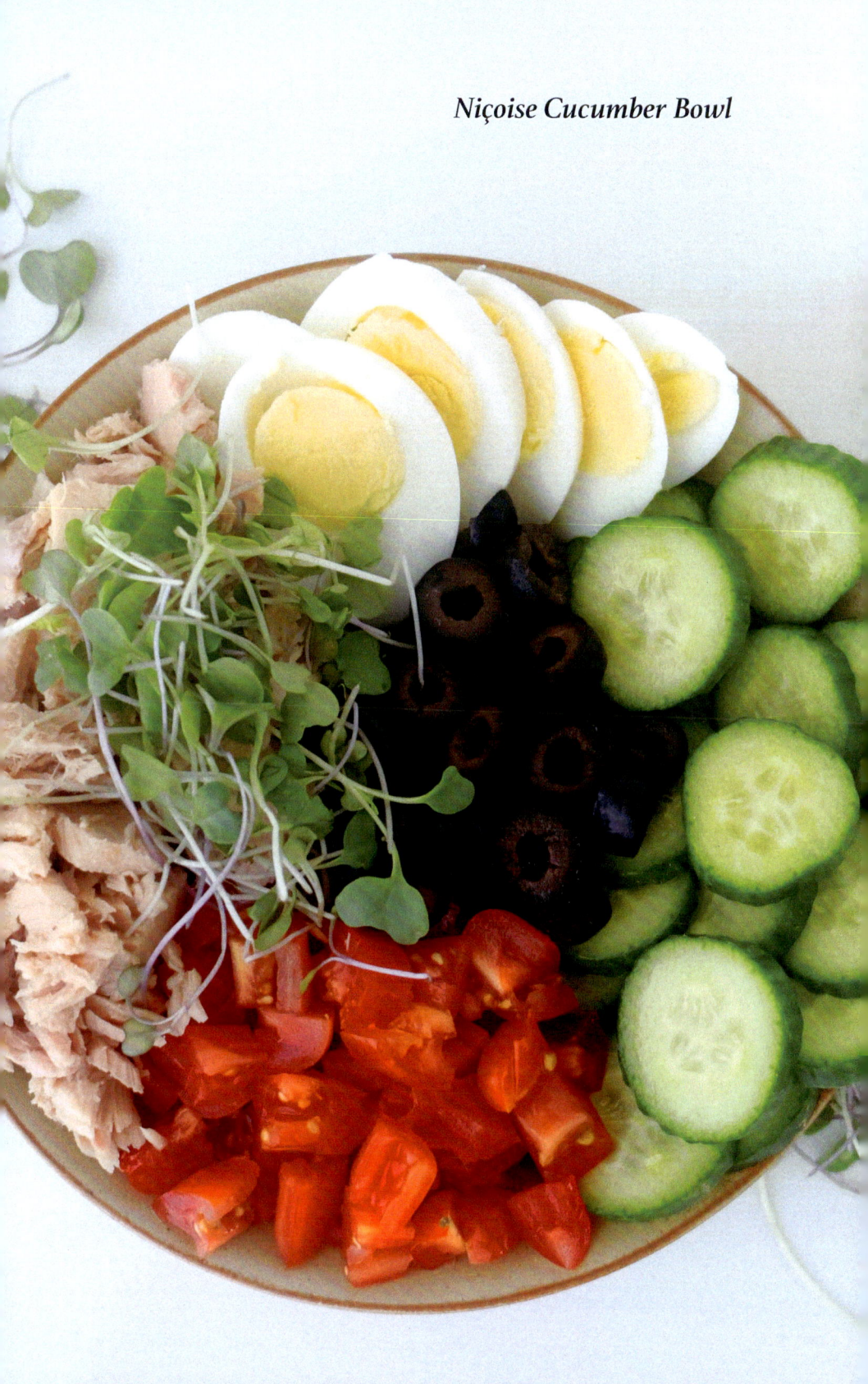

Niçoise Cucumber Bowl

Sesame Ginger Cucumber Bowl

For this Asian inspired bowl, cabbage forms the base accompanied by colorful veggies, shrimp, brown rice, and sesame ginger dressing. **Calories: 308**

1 hydroponic cucumber, sliced

1 cup shredded green or red cabbage

1 carrot, grated

¼ cup red onion

¼ green onions

6 medium cooked shrimp

¼ cup cooked brown rice

2 Tbsp. low-fat sesame ginger dressing

1 Tbsp. sesame seeds

Directions: Put the shredded cabbage in a bowl, then top with cucumber, carrot, and red onion. Arrange cooked shrimp in bowl and sprinkle with ¼ cup cooked brown rice. Drizzle with sesame ginger dressing, then sprinkle with sesame seeds and green onions.

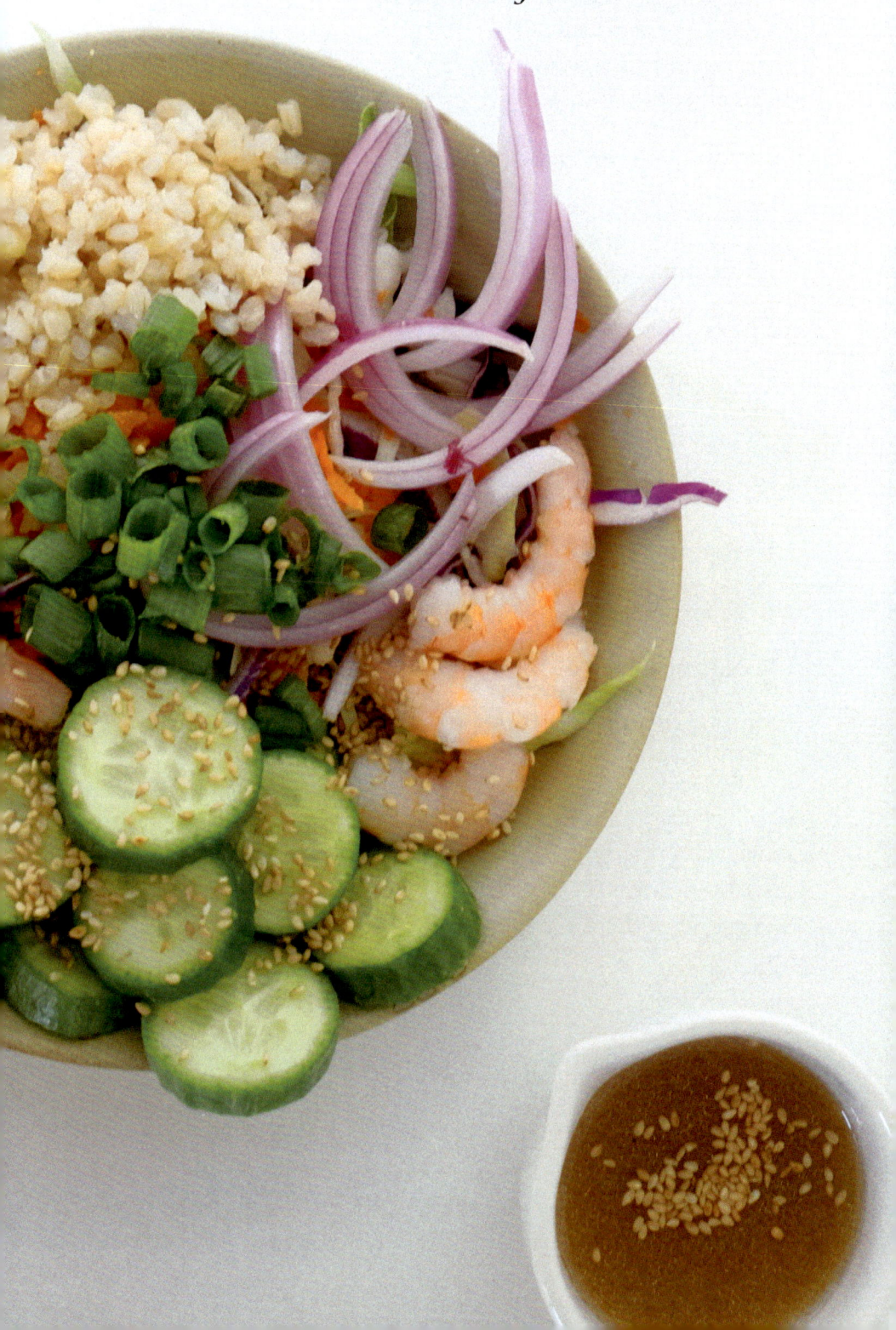

Sesame Ginger Cucumber Bowl

The Mediterranean Cucumber Bowl

Get a taste of the Mediterranean with this cucumber bowl that features bright flavors like lemon and is loaded with the healthy protein of chickpeas and sunflower seeds. **Calories: 355**

1 hydroponic cucumber, sliced

I Roma tomato, chopped

½ red onion, chopped

5 olives, sliced

½ cup chickpeas

1 Tbsp. sunflower seeds

¼ cup cooked quinoa

2 Tbsp. balsamic dressing

1 radish, sliced

¼ cup chopped parsley and mint

Squeeze or splash of lemon juice

Directions: Toss chopped cucumber, tomato, red onion, and olives together. Add chickpeas, radishes, and quinoa, then sprinkle with sunflower seeds. Drizzle with balsamic dressing, a dash of lemon juice, and sprinkle with parsley and mint.

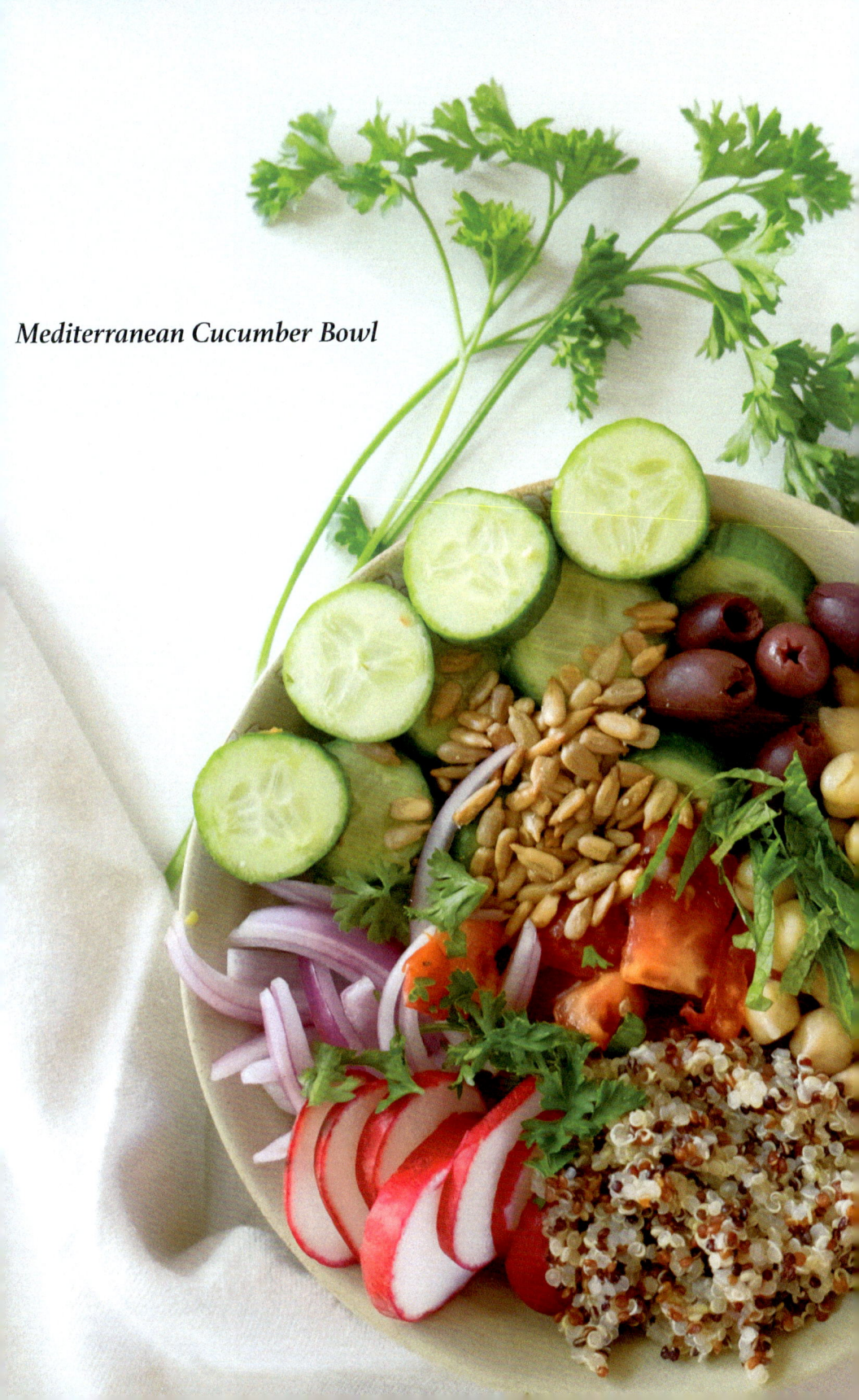

Mediterranean Cucumber Bowl

The Italian Cucumber Bowl

This mix of salami, pepperoncini, and parmesan is going to keep you satisfied without all the extra fat and calories. **Calories: 420**

1 hydroponic cucumber, sliced

½ head of romaine lettuce, chopped

Handful of grape or cherry tomatoes

5 kalamata olives

1 pepperoncino, chopped

3 thick slices salami, chopped

½ cup cooked lentils

2 Tbsp. parmesan

Light Italian dressing

¼ Italian parsley, chopped

Directions: Put romaine lettuce in bowl, then assemble chopped cucumber, and pepperoncino on top. Arrange tomatoes, olives, chopped or sliced salami, and lentils in the bowl. Drizzle with Italian dressing, then sprinkle with parmesan and parsley.

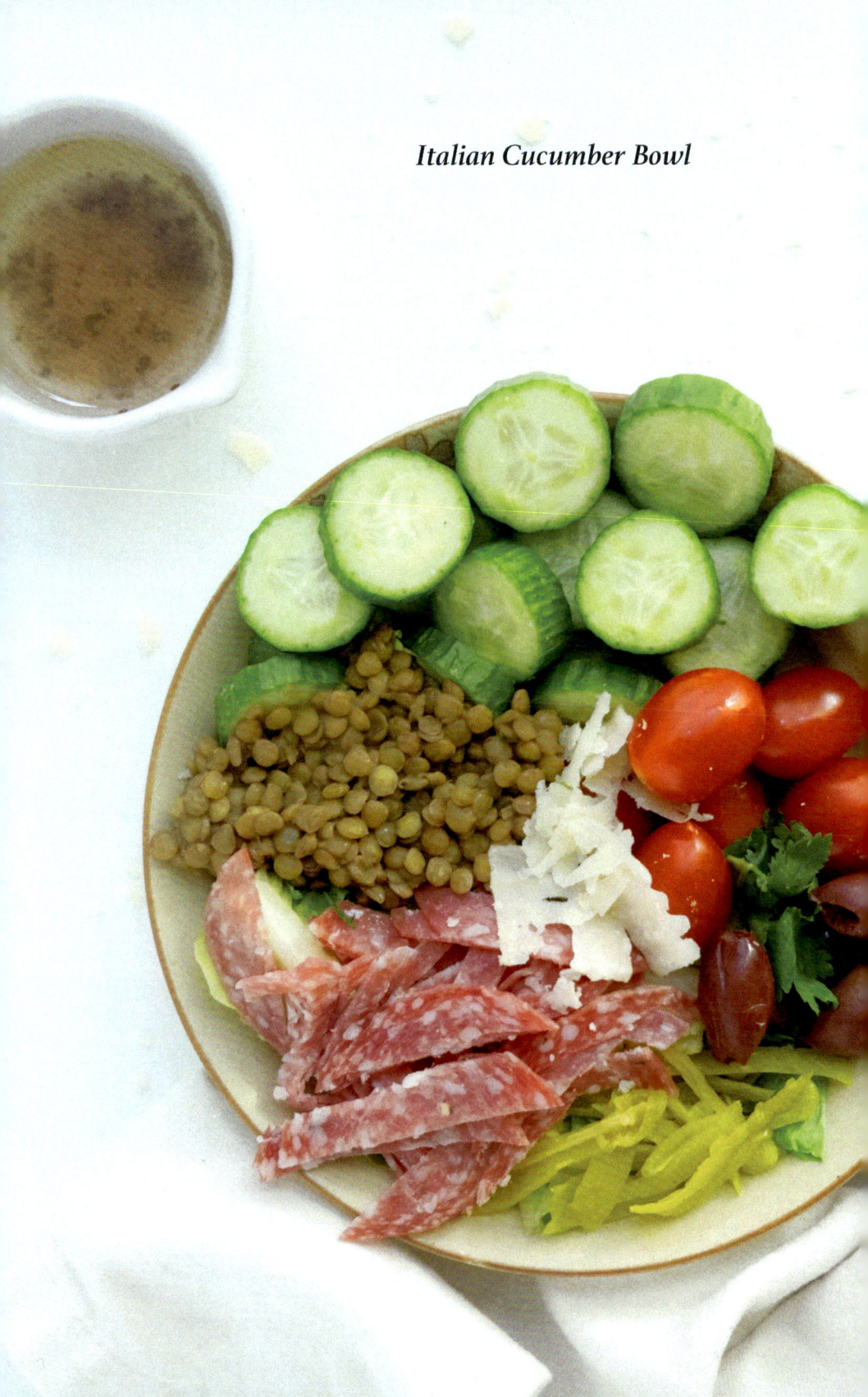

Italian Cucumber Bowl

The Cucumber Cobb Bowl

A take on the traditional Cobb, this simple bowl goes big with eggs, ham, and cottage cheese for a hearty but healthy meal. **Calories: 386**

1 hydroponic cucumber, sliced

1 cup spinach

1 beefsteak or Roma tomato, sliced

¼ cup green onions

1 slice of ham, cut thick and chopped

1 hardboiled egg, sliced

¼ of an avocado sliced

Light Catalina dressing

Directions: Fill the bottom of the bowl with spinach, then layer the cucumber, tomato, and avocado slices. Sprinkle with chopped ham and green onions, then drizzle with Catalina dressing.

Getting a little too generous with your pour? These bowls are packed with flavor, so it's not necessary to drown ingredients in dressing. To avoid the dreaded overpour, remember that two tablespoons is about one ounce. You know what else is just over an ounce? Most standard shot glasses. Dig yours out from the back of the cupboard and put it to good use.

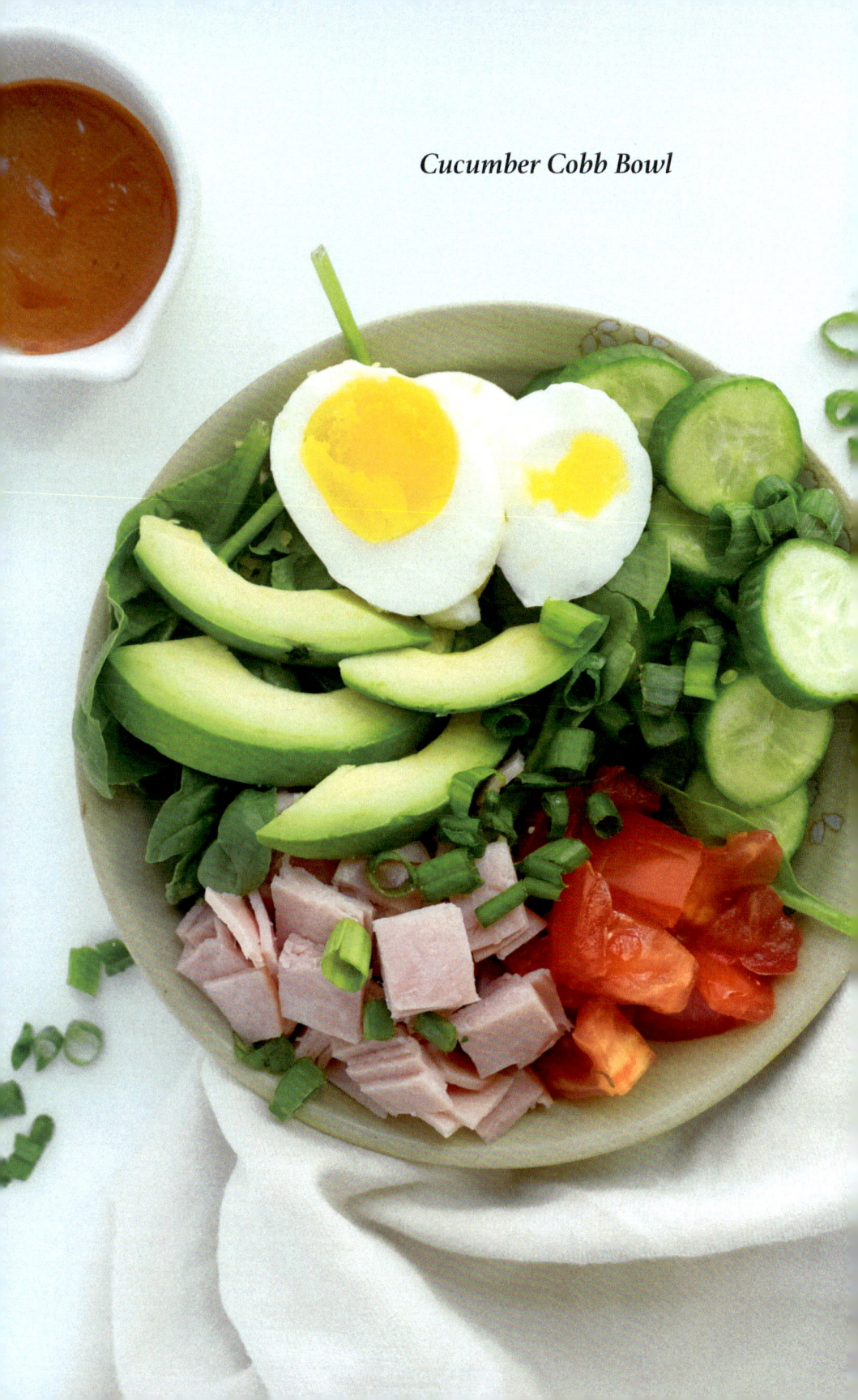

Cucumber Cobb Bowl

The Moroccan Cucumber Bowl

Get a taste of the exotic with our Moroccan cucumber bowl featuring tempeh, chickpeas and a punch of mint. **Calories: 410**

1 hydroponic cucumber, sliced

1 carrot, shredded

1 tomato, chopped

¼ cup green onions

¼ cup tempeh

½ cup chickpeas

¼ cup cooked quinoa

Lemon mint vinaigrette:

2 Tbsp. lemon juice

½ Tbsp. extra-virgin olive oil

1 Tbsp. vinegar

¼ cup fresh mint

Directions: Prepare vegetables. Toss cucumber, carrot, quinoa and tomato in a bowl. Top with cubed or sliced tempeh and chickpeas. Drizzle with dressing and sprinkle with green onions.

For the lemon mint vinaigrette: Put lemon juice, extra-virgin olive oil, vinegar, and mint into a food processor and pulse until desired consistency. Keep refrigerated.

Alternate salad dressing: Light balsamic vinaigrette

Moroccan Cucumber Bowl

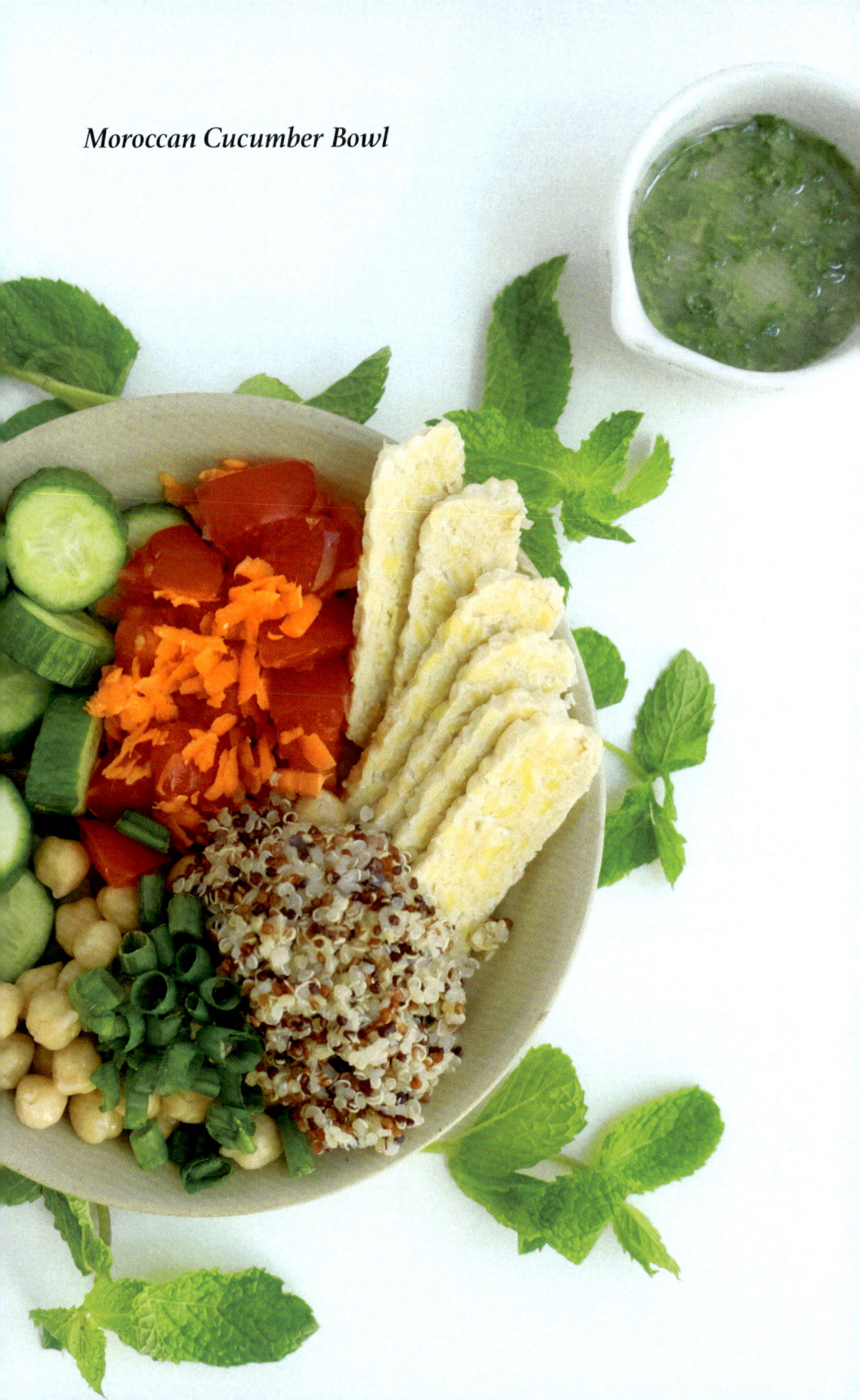

Big Greek Cucumber Bowl

Go Greek with big, bold flavors like kalamata olives, sardines, and feta cheese. **Calories: 369**

1 hydroponic cucumber, sliced

2 Roma tomatoes, chopped

1 bell pepper, diced or sliced

5 kalamata olives, whole or sliced

1 sardine

½ cup chickpeas

2 Tbsp. crumbled feta

2 Tbsp. light balsamic vinaigrette

¼ cup parsley

Directions: Toss cucumber, tomatoes, bell pepper, and olives together in a bowl. Top with sardine and chickpeas, then sprinkle with feta. Drizzle with vinaigrette, then sprinkle with chopped parsley.

A word of warning about canned fish…One of the things that can quickly tip your calorie count is to inadvertently use sardines or tuna packed in oil instead of water. While the oil does keep the fish moist and flavorful, it also adds calories and cholesterol. Opt for water packed sardines and let your salad dressing carry the flavor in this cucumber bowl.

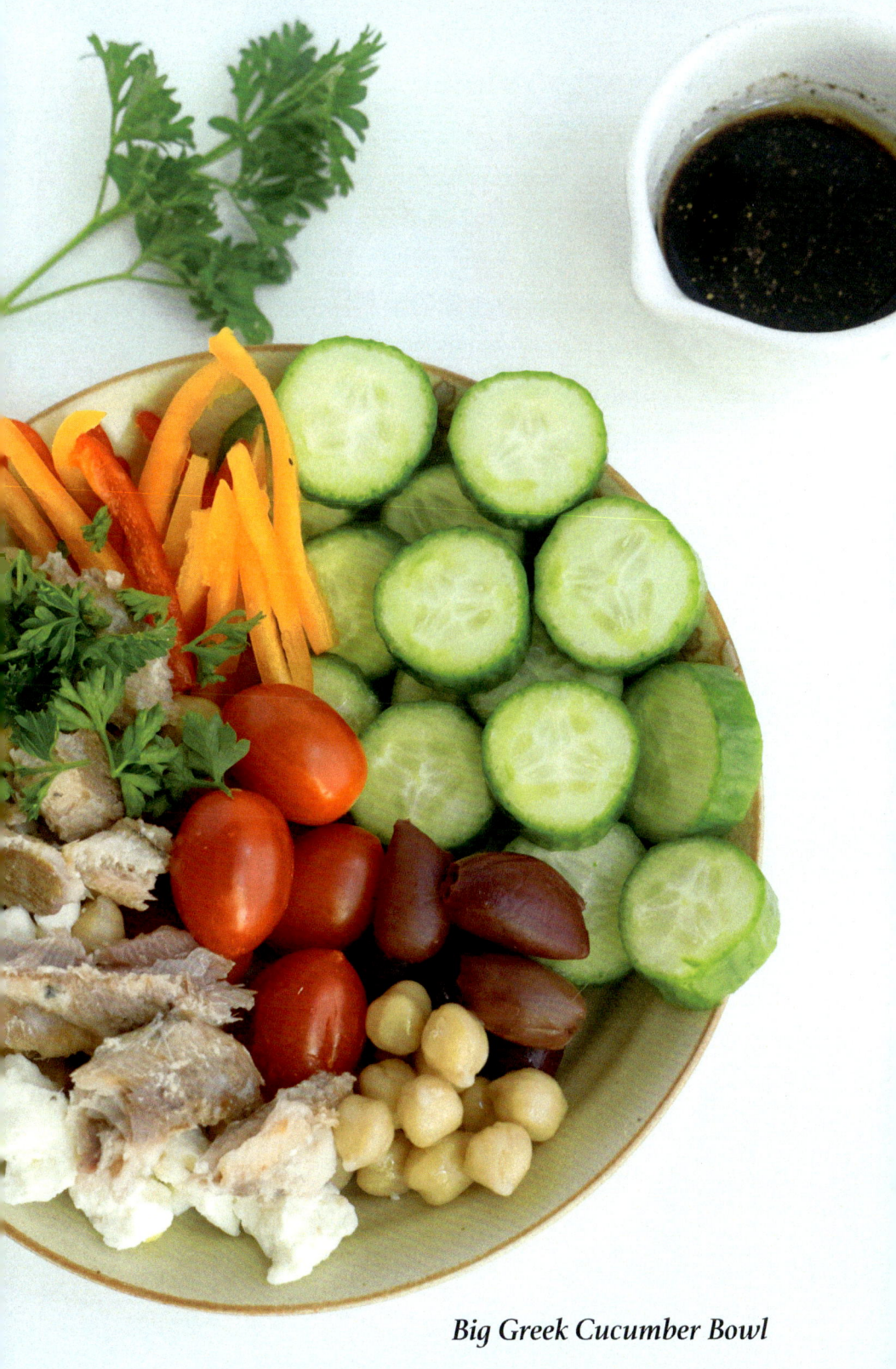

Big Greek Cucumber Bowl

Other Bowl Options

Getting bored? Start mixing and matching to discover your own favorite flavors. Use the grid to create a cucumber bowl that stays within your recommended calorie range but still includes all your favorite things. Here are a few ideas you can use to spark your sense of culinary adventure.

Big Vegan Cucumber Bowl: Cucumber, Cauliflower, Broccoli, Carrots, Mushrooms, Tofu, Lentils, Quinoa, Balsamic vinaigrette

Meat Lovers Bowl: Cucumber, Lettuce, Onions, Tomato, Bell Pepper, Roast Beef, Ham, Cheddar, Fat-free Catalina Dressing, Salt & Pepper

Lebanese Cucumber Bowl: Cucumber, Red Onion, Chickpeas, Kidney Beans, Quinoa, Avocado oil, Lemon juice, Dill and Mint

Build Your Own Chart
Start with one whole large cucumber sliced 47 cal WOMEN MEN

CATEGORY A		PICK 3	PICK 3
Carrot	30 cal/carrot		
Broccoli	34 cal/head of broccoli		
Tomato	18 cal/tomato		
Onion	30 cal/half onion		
Bell Pepper	24 cal/bell pepper		
Spinach	23 cal/cup		
Cauliflower	31 cal/head of cauliflower		
Olives	25 cal/5 olives		
Cabbage	17 cal/1 cup shredded		

CATEGORY B		PICK 2	PICK 3
Tuna	100 cal/can		
Tofu	100 cal/serving		
Ham	105 cal/3 slices		
Chicken	75 cal/3 slices		
Turkey	75 cal/3 slices		
Roast Beef	90 cal/3 slices		
Tempeh	80 cal/4th cup		
Sardines	71 cal/1 sardine		
Black Beans	110 cal/half cup		
Chickpeas	105 cal/half cup		
Kidney Bean	105 cal/half cup		
Lentils	110 cal/half cup		
Hard Boiled Egg	78 cal/egg		
Shrimp	48 cal/6 medium		

CATEGORY C		PICK 1	PICK 2
Cottage Cheese	20 cal/2 tbsp		
Feta	34 cal/2 tbsp		
Parmesan	40 cal/2 tbsp		
Aged Cheddar	43 cal/2 tbsp		
Mozzarella	31 cal/2 tbsp		
Quinoa	55 cal/4th cup		
Avocado	35 cal/4th slice of avocado		
Brown Rice	50 cal/4th cup		

CATEGORY D		PICK 1	PICK 1
Balsamic Dressing	28 cal/2 tbsp		
Light Balsamic Vinaigrette	45 cal/2 tbsp		
Light Italian	60 cal/2 tbsp		
Fat-Free Catalina	50 cal/2 tbsp		
Low-Fat Sesame Ginger	35 cal/2 tbsp		
EVCO	60 cal/half tbsp		
Avocado Oil	60 cal/half tbsp		
MCT Oil	65 cal/half tbsp		

FREEBIES - Unlimited
Lemon/Lime Squeeze / Hot Sauce / Salt and Pepper / Herbs and Spices / Cilantro, Basil, and All Lettuces / Radish / Capers / Mushrooms / Celery / Vinegar

Dinner is Served

When you're on a diet, one of the difficulties that can derail you is the dilemma of having to cook for a crowd. If you have to make one meal for your family and another for yourself, the logistics involved can quickly sabotage the best of intentions. That's why the Cucumber Diet has a wide variety of flexible, delicious recipes so you can serve up something everyone will be excited about with a focus on fresh ingredients you can find at any grocery store.

Most of the dinner recipes can be made in 20-30 minutes from start to finish, including prep and cook time. Not everyone, however, has time to make a meal from scratch. At the end of this section, you'll find some quick solutions for days when the schedule gets too hectic, so you can still stick to the plan and avoid the high caloric cost of takeout.

The recipes below are built to serve four and each serving clocks in at around 400 calories, but with the caveat that your dinner is a two-course meal. That's right- you get extras. Each dinner starts with a build-your-own half cucumber bowl. Just start with a cucumber and toss in two add-ins of your choice from the grid, one from column A and another from column B, topped with a dressing for a caloric cost of around 150 calories. The bonus of starting with some greenery is that it gets you full on the good stuff before you dig into the higher caloric density proteins and grains you'll find on most dinner plates.

Got dietary concerns or a vegan in the house? No problem. You'll find plenty of options to satisfy even the trickiest palate in our vegetarian section, most of them with ingredients you won't have to struggle to track down.

A word about dinner preparation

It's so essential that you don't eyeball ingredients that it's worth saying again. Don't trust yourself to be able to determine serving sizes or measurements. One tablespoon is just that—one level (not heaping) tablespoon. It's not just an exercise to limit your caloric intake. It's critical to learning conscious eating habits that will last you a lifetime.

Also, beware of substitutions. While it might be tempting to throw whatever you have in the pantry into the pot, it'll alter the calorie count for that meal significantly. Take for example the difference between black beans and refried beans. You might assume they are roughly equivalent, but one cup of black beans is about 100 calories while one cup of refried beans is 190 calories.

And finally, have fun. From tahini to golden raisins, now is the time to experiment with new flavors that bring a lot to the table without the high caloric cost.

Half Cucumber Bowl

This dressed down version of a cucumber bowl will prepare your palate for dinner and help you feel satisfied.

1 hydroponic cucumber, sliced

Choose your own add-in from column A in the build-your-own chart

Choose your own add-in from column B in the build-your-own chart

2 Tbsp. dressing of your choice

Your half cucumber bowl is a flexible way to get in extra fiber and veggies. Simply pair your favorite mix-ins from the cucumber grid for lunch and drizzle with dressing. No matter which way you slice it, you'll come in under 150 calories.

Trout with Orange and White Wine Couscous

Got fresh fish? Then we've got a treat on the line for you. Trout infused with white wine and citrus. **Calories: 408**

- **2 tablespoons 2% reduced-fat Greek yogurt**

- **2 tablespoons chopped fresh chives**

- **2 tablespoons olive oil, divided**

- **4 teaspoons orange juice, divided**

- **4 (6-ounce) trout fillets**

- **1 1/8 teaspoons kosher salt, divided**

- **1/2 teaspoon black pepper, divided**

- **1 cup finely chopped carrots**

- **1 cup finely chopped zucchini**

- **1/4 cup minced shallots**

- **2 teaspoons minced garlic**

- **1/3 cup dry white wine**

- **1 cup cooked couscous**

Directions: *Heat oven to 450 degrees. Combine yogurt, chives, 2 tsp. oil, and one tablespoon orange juice in a bowl. Whisk until smooth. Sprinkle fish with salt and pepper to taste, then rub with yogurt mixture. Heat ovenproof skillet on high heat. Put 1 tsp. oil in the pan. Add fish, skin side down, and cook 2-3 minutes. Transfer skillet to oven and bake at 450 degrees for five minutes. Turn fish halfway through.*

Heat a separate skillet on medium-high heat. Add remaining 1 tablespoon oil to the pan. Add carrots, shallots, and garlic; cook 4 minutes, stirring occasionally. Add zucchini and remaining 1 teaspoon orange juice, remaining salt, pepper, and wine. Cook 30 seconds. Add couscous and toss.

Serve fish with on bed of vegetable couscous.

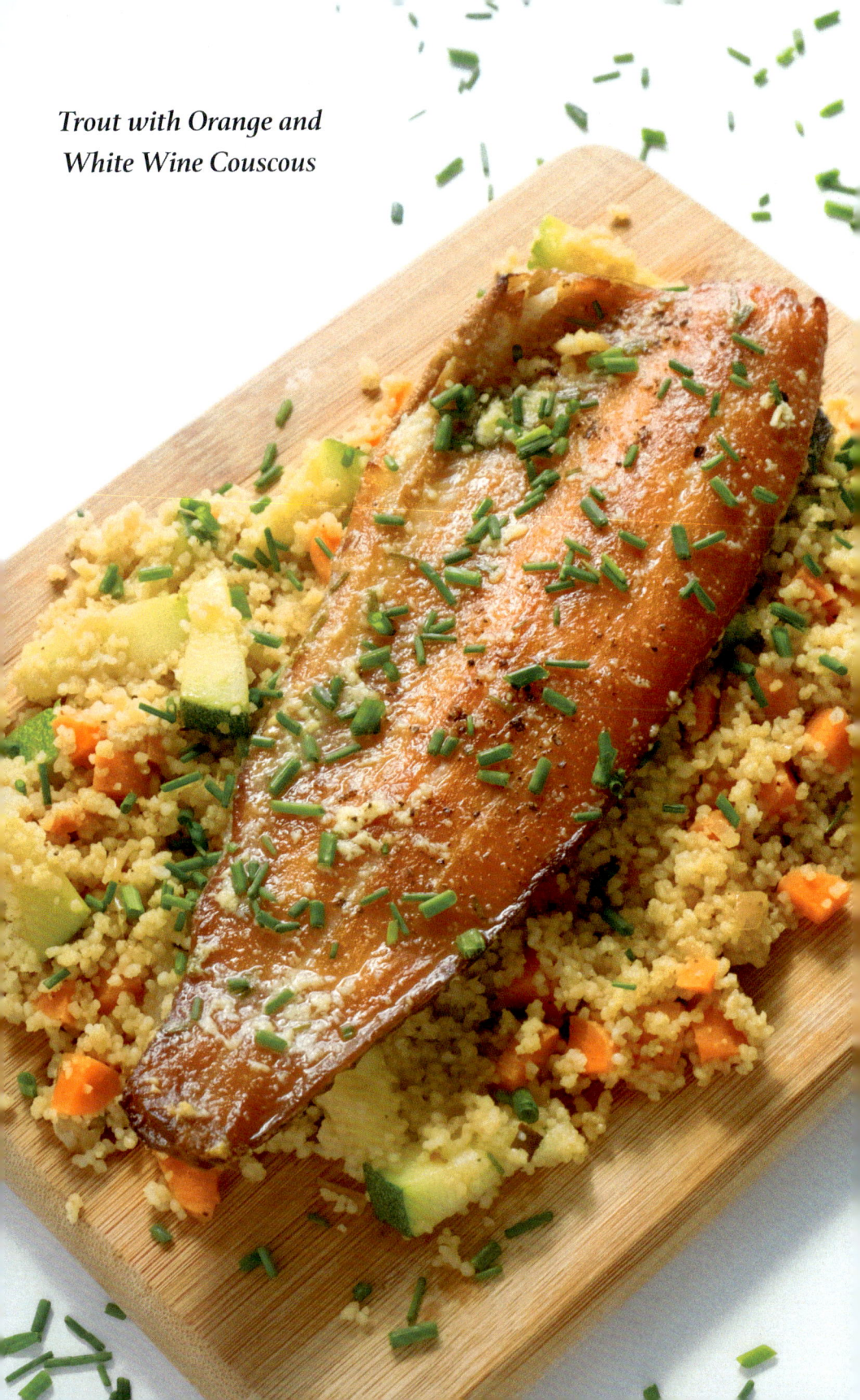

Trout with Orange and White Wine Couscous

Moroccan Salmon with Cauliflower

This eastern-inspired dish takes the flavors of salmon and cauliflower and infuses spice and a touch of sweetness. **Calories: 422**

1 tablespoon olive oil

1 teaspoon ground curry, divided

3/4 teaspoon kosher salt, divided

1/8 teaspoon freshly ground black pepper

4 cups cauliflower florets

1/4 cup chopped fresh cilantro

1/4 cup golden or regular raisins

1 tablespoon fresh lime juice

1/2 teaspoon ground coriander

1/8 teaspoon ground allspice

4 (4 1/2-oz.) salmon fillets (about 1 in. thick)

Cooking spray

4 lime wedges

Directions: *Preheat oven to 450 degrees. Combine olive oil, ½ tsp. curry, salt, and pepper in a large bowl, then add cauliflower and toss. Arrange cauliflower in a single layer on a baking sheet. Bake at 450 18-20 minutes until brown. Mix cooked cauliflower with raisins, cilantro, and lime juice, tossing to combine.*

Reduce oven heat to 400. Combine remaining curry, ½ tsp. salt, coriander, and all-spice in a small bowl. Rub the mixture onto the curry filets. Arrange on a foiled lined baking sheet coated with cooking spray. Cook at 400 degrees for 10 minutes. Serve with cooked cauliflower and lime wedges.

Dill Tilapia with Asparagus

The tangy accents of lemon and dill highlight white fish in this quick and healthy meal for the grill. **Calories: 442**

4 tilapia fillets

2 tablespoons unsalted butter

1/4 cup chopped fresh dill

1/2 teaspoon kosher salt

1/2 teaspoon black pepper

8 lemon slices

2 tablespoons olive oil

1-pound asparagus

1 cup cooked quinoa

Cooking spray

Directions: *Heat grill to medium-high. Cut four pieces of foil twice as large as the tilapia filets and coat them with cooking spray. Top each fillet with 1 ½ tsp. butter and 1 tablespoon of dill. Top with salt, pepper, and lemon slices. Fold foil over and seal the packets of fish. Place on the grill 10-12 minutes, turning once halfway through.*

Combine olive oil and asparagus in a bowl and toss. Throw on the grill next to the fish packets for five minutes or until tender. Plate fish on top of a bed of ¼ cup quinoa and asparagus, then top with grilled lemon slices.

Garlic & Lime Butter Shrimp with Zoodles

A bright burst of lime and the decadence of butter is all shrimp needs to steal the show. Don't have to time spiralize zucchini? Just buy pre-packaged zoodles at the grocery store. **Calories: 427**

2 tablespoons unsalted butter

2 tablespoons extra-virgin olive oil

3 garlic cloves

Zest and juice of 1 lime

⅓ cup dry white wine

1½ pounds large tail-on shrimp, peeled

Kosher salt and freshly ground black pepper

3 pounds zucchini, spiralized

Lime wedges, as needed for serving

⅓ cup chopped fresh parsley

Directions: *In a large skillet on medium heat, melt the butter. Add olive oil and garlic and cook until fragrant. Add lime zest, juice, and wine. Bring to simmer until liquid is reduced, about 3 minutes. Add shrimp and sauté another three minutes. Season with salt and pepper. Remove from skillet.*

Add zucchini to the skillet and season with salt and pepper. Stir and cook until tender, about 5 minutes. Return the shrimp to the pan and toss. Serve with lime wedges and parsley.

By Land

Simple Soy Beef Stir-Fry

Whipping up this simple stir-fry from the leftovers in your fridge is a lot easier than you might think. Don't have beef? Use chicken instead and get fewer calories into the bargain. **Calories: 462**

2 tablespoons sesame oil, divided

10 ounces flank steak, thinly sliced

1/2 teaspoon black pepper

1/4 teaspoon kosher salt

1/4 cup dark brown sugar

3 tablespoons reduced-sodium soy sauce

2 tablespoons unseasoned rice vinegar

3 cups fresh zucchini

3 cups sliced red bell peppers (about 2 medium)

1 cup hot cooked brown rice

1/2 cup chopped green onions

Directions: *Heat sesame oil in a large skillet or wok on high. Salt and pepper flank steak slices, then add to skillet and cook until browned. Remove from skillet.*

Combine brown sugar, soy sauce, and vinegar in a small bowl. Add the remaining tablespoon of sesame oil, zucchini and bell peppers to the skillet or wok you used to cook the steak. Cover and steam on high 2 minutes. Uncover and add soy sauce mixture. Cook 5-6 minutes until liquid reduces by half but vegetables are still crisp. Add steak, stir and serve over ¼ cup rice. Top with green onions.

5-minute Chicken Quesadillas

Pressed for time? Pick up a rotisserie chicken and try these quick quesadillas. **Calories: 448**

1 tablespoon olive oil

4 teaspoons all-purpose flour

1/2 cup unsalted chicken stock

1 cup coarsely chopped spinach

1 tablespoon hot sauce (optional)

1/4 teaspoon kosher salt

1/8 teaspoon black pepper

½ of a boneless rotisserie chicken, shredded

4 ounces mozzarella cheese, shredded

4 small whole-wheat flour tortillas (8-inches)

Cooking spray

Directions: *Heat oil in a saucepan on medium-high. Sprinkle flour over oil and cook 30 seconds, stirring constantly. Slowly add stock, cook 2 minutes until thick. Remove from pan. Stir in spinach, hot sauce, salt and pepper, chicken, and shredded cheese.*

Heat a skillet on medium. Divide chicken evenly over four tortillas, putting it on one side of the tortilla. Fold tortillas over. Coat heated skillet with cooking spray, add quesadillas to skillet and brown on each side until cheese is melted. Cut into wedges.

Bruce's Bolognese

This classic recipe gets a healthy face-lift with chicken and fresh carrots.

Calories: 484

8 oz. linguine or fettuccine

4 tsp. olive oil

1 lb. ground chicken breast

salt and pepper

2 medium carrots

2 medium stalks celery

1 large onion

1 clove garlic

1 can crushed tomatoes

1/2 c. reduced-fat (2%) milk

4 oz. freshly grated Parmesan cheese

1/4 c. loosely packed fresh parsley leaves

Directions: *Heat large covered saucepot of salted water to boiling on high. Add pasta and cook as label directs. Meanwhile, in a 12-inch nonstick skillet, heat 2 teaspoons oil on medium 1 minute. Add ground chicken to skillet; sprinkle with 1/4 teaspoon salt. Cook chicken 8 to 9 minutes, or until it is no longer pink, stirring occasionally. Transfer chicken along with any juices in skillet to medium bowl.*

To the same skillet, add remaining 2 teaspoons oil with carrots, celery, onion, and garlic; cook 10 to 12 minutes or until vegetables are lightly browned and tender, stirring occasionally. Stir in tomatoes, 1/4 teaspoon salt, and 1/4 teaspoon freshly ground black pepper; heat to boiling. Reduce heat to medium-low and simmer, uncovered, 10 minutes, stirring occasionally. Stir in cooked chicken and milk; heat through.

Reserve 1/4 cup pasta cooking water. Drain pasta and return to saucepot; stir in the sauce from skillet, Parmesan, parsley, and reserved cooking water, and toss to coat.

Peruvian Steak Bowl

A little sweet potato, pumpkin seeds, and a drizzle of honey lime sauce make this spicy bowl a surefire hit with the fam. Make the ingredients ahead for quick assembly. **Calories: 507**

1 cup cooked brown rice1/4 salsa verde

1 cup cubed roasted sweet potato

6 ounces grilled flank steak, sliced

2 Tbsp. roasted pumpkin seed kernels

¼ cup fresh cilantro

Honey-Lime Sauce:

1 Tbsp. olive oil

1 Tbsp. honey

1 teaspoon fresh lime juice

Directions: *Combine cooked rice and salsa verde, then de into four bowls. Top each bowl with roasted sweet potato, sliced grilled flank steak, pumpkin seeds, and cilantro. Whisk together the olive oil, honey, and fresh lime juice and drizzle over the steak bowls.*

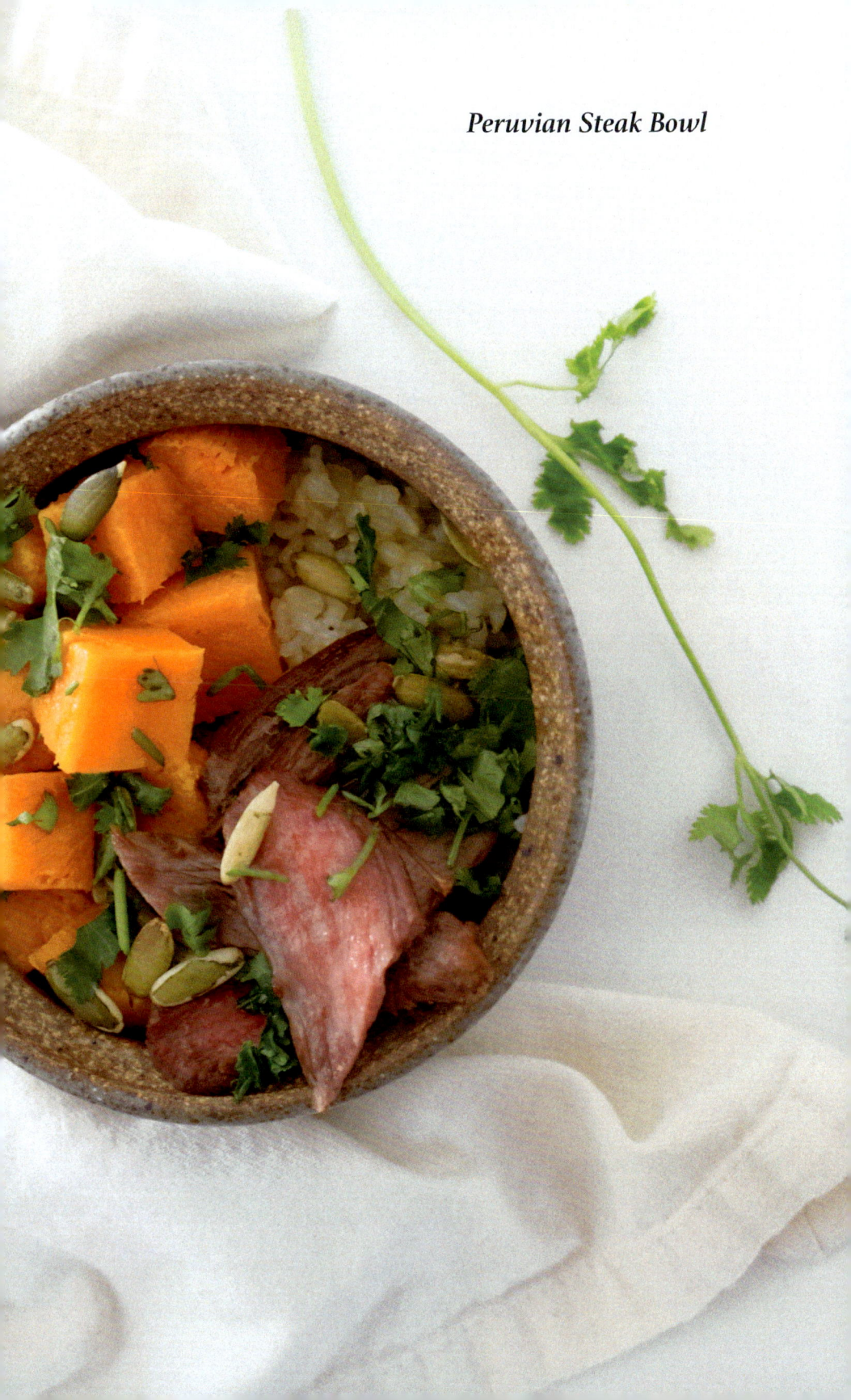

Peruvian Steak Bowl

Smoked Pork Tenderloin with Apples & Sweet Potatoes

Apples and sweet potatoes make the perfect partners to this paprika and cumin crusted pork. **Calories: 413**

- 1 (1-pound) pork tenderloin, trimmed
- 2 teaspoons smoked paprika
- 3/4 teaspoon kosher salt, divided
- 1/2 teaspoon freshly ground black pepper
- 1/2 teaspoon ground cumin
- 2 tablespoons olive oil, divided
- 2 large sweet potatoes, peeled and cut into 8 wedges each
- 1 ½ cups sliced apples (about 2 apples with skin on)
- 1/4 cup cider vinegar
- 3 tablespoons honey
- 1 teaspoon Dijon mustard
- 2 rosemary sprigs
- 1 tablespoon unsalted butter

Directions: *Heat oven to 350. Combine paprika, ¼ tsp. salt, pepper, and cumin in a small bowl. Rub the spices onto the pork tenderloin. Heat skillet on medium-high, adding 1 Tablespoon of oil to the pan. Add pork, cooking 8 minutes and turning halfway through to brown both sides.*

Put sweet potatoes and apples on a baking sheet, drizzling with1 tablespoon oil. Bake at 450° for 10 minutes. Stir potatoes and apples, then add pork to pan. Bake at 450 degrees for 15 minutes or until a meat thermometer registers 140°. Remove from oven. Sprinkle potatoes and apples with remaining salt. Let stand 5 minutes before cutting pork.

While you're waiting, combine vinegar, honey, mustard, and thyme in a small saucepan and bring to a boil. Cook 3 minutes, then add butter, stirring until melted. Remove rosemary sprigs and discard. Drizzle mixture over potatoes and apples. Serve with pork.

Cheddar & Parmesan Bacon Risotto

A combination of cheeses will make this hearty, fragrant risotto a family favorite. **Calories: 405**

4 cups chicken stock

2 cloves garlic, minced

2 bacon slices

1 1/4 cups diced onion

1 cup Arborio rice

1/2 cup dry white wine

1/4 teaspoon kosher salt

1/2 teaspoon black pepper

1 cup frozen green peas, thawed

1 teaspoon finely chopped fresh parsley

1/3 cup cheddar cheese, shredded

1/3 cup parmesan cheese

1/4 cup chopped parsley

Directions: *Bring chicken stock and garlic to a simmer over low heat. Cook bacon slices in a large skillet, then cool and crumble. In the same skillet, sauté the onion until brown. Add the rice, cooking one minute or until fragrant. Add wine, cooking until liquid is absorbed. Stir in stock a cup at a time, stirring frequently and waiting until it is slowly absorbed before adding more. Reserve ¼ cup of stock. Stir salt and pepper, peas, chopped parsley, and cheese into the rice. Remove from heat and stir in reserved stock. Divide into four bowls and top with bacon and ¼ cup chopped parsley.*

Gouda Kale Beef Sliders

Open wide cause this recipe is a mouthful you'll want to make room for on your dinner plate. **Calories: 393, Serving size 2 sliders**

7 ounces kale, trimmed

1 1/2 tablespoons white wine vinegar

1 tablespoon extra-virgin olive oil

1 teaspoon sugar

1-pound lean ground sirloin

1 teaspoon smoked paprika

1/2 teaspoon Worcestershire sauce

1/4 teaspoon kosher salt

1/4 teaspoon freshly ground black pepper

4 slices reduced-fat gouda cheese

8 whole-wheat slider buns

Cooking spray

Directions: *Heat skillet over medium heat, coating with cooking spray. Add kale and cook 5 minutes until softened. Combine vinegar, oil, and sugar in a bowl and toss cooked kale. Set aside.*

Combine beef, paprika, Worcestershire, salt and pepper in a bowl. Shape into 8 small patties. Coat the same skillet you cooked the kale in with more cooking spray. Add patties. Cook 2-3 minutes turning halfway. Top with half a slice of cheese, cover, and cook another minute or so until the cheese melts. Place patty on bun, top with kale.

Broccoli Gnocchi

Can you really make your own gnocchi from veggies? You betcha. This recipe uses broccoli stalks in place of potatoes. **Calories: 437**

3 cups broccoli florets

1 cup parmesan grated

2 egg yolks

1 tsp garlic powder

1/2 tsp salt

1/4 tsp pepper

1 tsp xanthan gum

3/4 cup coconut flour

12 oz mozzarella cheese

2 Tbsp. butter

2 cloves garlic, minced

¼ cup torn fresh basil leaves

Directions: *Steam broccoli until tender. Cool. Use a food processor to mash until smooth. Add remaining ingredients except for mozzarella into the food processor. Pulse until combined. Place mozzarella cheese in a small bowl and microwave 1-2 minutes until melted. Stir into broccoli mixture until combined. Wet fingers and form 48 gnocchi using 1-2 Tbsp. of batter per gnocchi. Crimp with fork and place on a baking sheet in freezer for up to one hour.*

Bring a large pot of salted water to a boil. Place 10-12 gnocchi in the boiling water for 1-2 minutes at a time. Drain. Melt 2 Tbsp. butter and minced garlic together in a skillet. Sauté cooked gnocchi briefly in skillet and top with fresh basil.

Meatball & Mushroom Fondue

This family favorite is like a cross between stroganoff and traditional meatballs with plenty of opportunities for dipping across the table.
Calories: 471

3/4 cup shredded yellow squash

10 ounces ground turkey

1/3 cup diced red onion

1/2 teaspoon dried oregano

1/4 teaspoon kosher salt

1/4 teaspoon black pepper

1 large egg

1 tablespoon olive oil

8 ounces sliced shitake or Baby Bella mushrooms

2 garlic cloves, minced

1 1/2 cups marinara sauce

1/4 cup water

4 ounces part-skim mozzarella cheese, shredded

4 ounces whole-wheat baguette, cut into 24 thin slices and toasted

¼ cup chopped Italian parsley

Cooking spray

Directions: *Heat oven to 400. Line a baking sheet with foil, then coat with cooking spray. Squeeze extra moisture from shredded yellow squash by placing it between two paper towels. Stir squash, turkey, onion, oregano, salt, pepper, and egg into a bowl. Form 24 meatballs about ¾-1 Tbsp in diameter each. Bake at 400 degrees on baking sheet until cooked, about 10-12 minutes.*

Add oil to an ovenproof skillet on medium-high, then add mushrooms and garlic, cooking until most liquid has evaporated about 5 minutes. Stir in marinara sauce and water, reduce heat and simmer another five minutes. Add cooked meatballs to the skillet and toss gently to coat with sauce. Sprinkle with cheese. Preheat broiler and toast skillet just until cheese is melted about 2 minutes. Serve with toasted bread for dipping and sprinkle with Italian parsley.

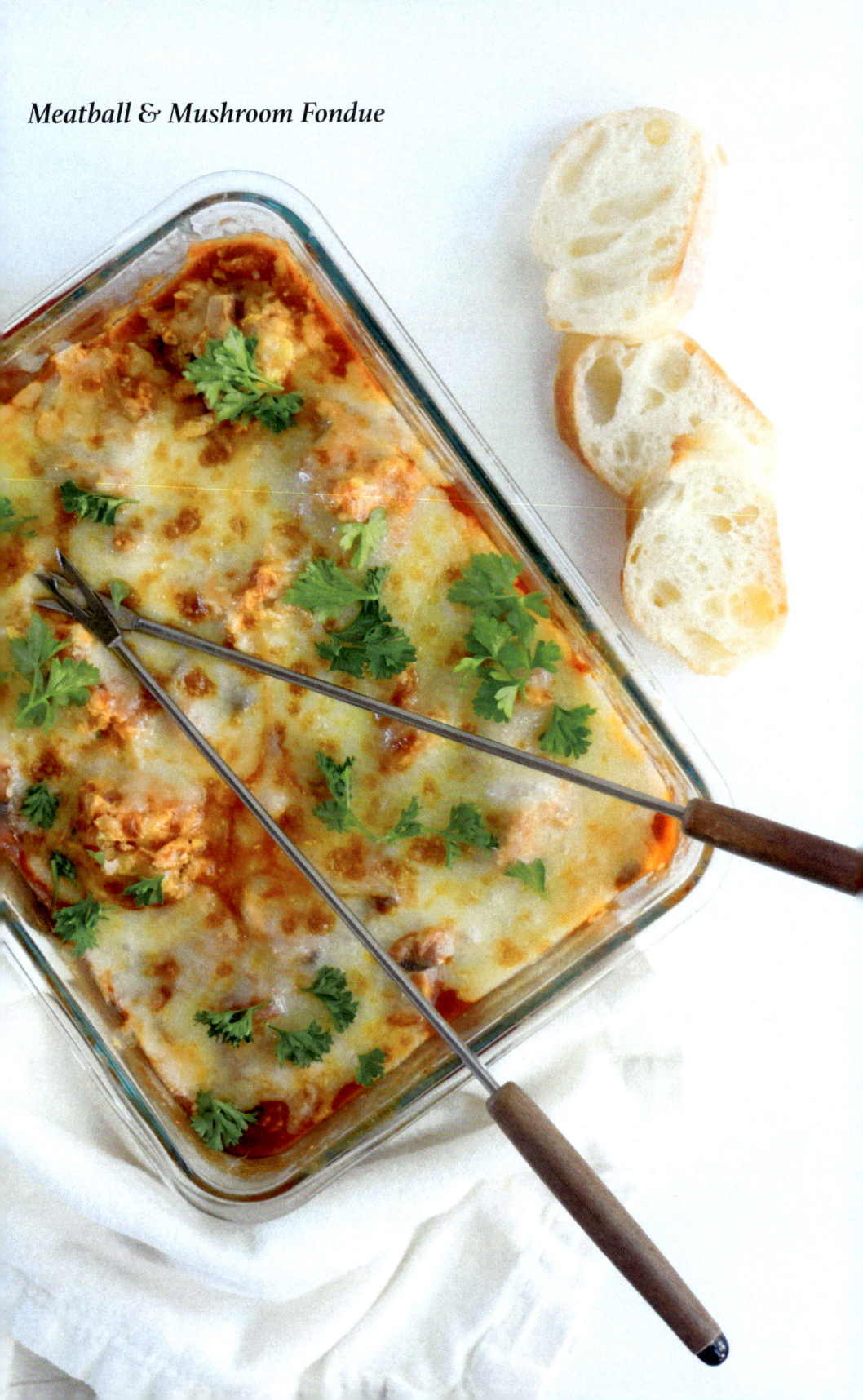

Meatball & Mushroom Fondue

Fresh Tomato Soup and Pita Chips

A comforting classic for a cold day, this recipe keeps it vegetarian with a side of savory pita chips. **Calories: 410**

For Soup

3 tbsp. olive oil

1 large onion

1/2 tsp. salt

2 cloves garlic, grated

1 1-inch piece ginger, grated

2 tsp. ground coriander

1 tsp. ground cumin

1 cup chopped red bell pepper

2 1/2 lb. fresh tomatoes, chopped

2 1/2 c. water

For Pita chips

4 pocketless pitas

2 tbsp. melted butter or olive oil

2 tbsp. cilantro

Directions: *In a Dutch oven or soup pot, heat olive oil on medium-low. Add onion, red bell pepper, and salt. Cook covered and occasionally stir for 8-10 minutes until peppers are tender.*

Grate garlic and ginger. Add to Dutch oven and cook one minute. Stir in spices and cook another minute until fragrant. Add tomatoes and water. Increase heat and bring to a boil, then turn down to medium-low and simmer, partially covered, for 10 minutes.

Preheat broiler and move top rack 8-10 inches away from heat. Brush pitas with melted butter or olive oil and cut into wedges. Put them on a baking sheet and sprinkle with cilantro. Toast 1-2 minutes or until slightly browned.

Using an immersion blender, puree soup until smooth. Serve with pita chips.

Smokey Vegetarian Chili

With a subtle kick from chipotles, this black-eyed pea-based chili is off-the-charts delicious. If you don't have a traditional pressure cooker, an Insta-pot works nicely for this recipe. **Calories: 452**

2 chipotles in adobo

2 cloves garlic

1/2 c. sun-dried tomatoes

1 (28 oz.) can whole peeled tomatoes

1 tbsp. oil

1 medium onion, chopped

1 medium green bell pepper, chopped

1 tbsp. chili powder

4 c. lower-sodium broth

2 c. black-eyed peas

1/2 tsp. salt

Avocado, for serving

Cheddar, shredded, for serving

Cilantro, for serving

Tortilla Chips, for serving

Directions: *In a food processor, puree chipotles and sun-dried tomatoes. Add tomatoes and pulse until chopped. In a pressure cooker or Instapot on medium, put oil, green bell pepper and chili powder into the pot. Add tomato mixture, black-eyed peas, and salt. Lock lid and cook under high pressure for 12-20 minutes. Release pressure. Serve bowls of chili with slices of avocado, cheddar cheese, cilantro, and a serving of tortilla chips.*

Eggplant Parm in a Hurry

Get this Italian favorite on the table in a hurry with this no-fuss recipe that sits on a bed of fresh spinach. **Calories: 401**

1/2 cup all-purpose flour

1 large egg plus 1 egg white

1 cup panko

1/2 cup freshly grated Parmesan cheese

1/2 tsp. garlic powder

Kosher salt and pepper

1 tbsp. olive oil

1 small eggplant (about 12 oz.)

2 cups fresh spinach

1 cup marinara sauce, warmed

½ cup shredded fresh mozzarella

Directions: *Preheat oven to 450°F. Line a baking sheet with foil. Put flour on a plate and beat the egg and egg white in a separate, shallow bowl. Combine panko, parmesan, garlic powder, salt and pepper in a pie plate or plate with high edges, then toss with oil*

Cut the eggplant into long 1/2-inch-thick slices. Coat slices in flour, then egg being sure to shake excess liquid off. Drop into the panko mixture, pressing to help it adhere. Transfer to the baking sheet and roast at 450 for 15 minutes or until brown.

Put fresh spinach at the bottom of a wide bowl or plate. Lay eggplant slices on top, top with large spoonfuls of marinara and mozzarella cheese.

Garden Minestrone Soup

A bowl that tastes like spring, this soup is overflowing with good stuff from the garden. **Calories: 437**

2 tbsp. olive oil

2 medium carrots, chopped

1 medium leek, thinly sliced

6 sprigs fresh thyme, tied together

Salt

2 large red potatoes, chopped

2-quart vegetable broth

1 bunch asparagus, sliced

1 can (15 oz.) navy beans, rinsed and drained

2 tbsp. chopped fresh basil

Directions: *In a large soup pot or Dutch oven, heat olive oil on medium. Add carrots, leek, fresh thyme, and 1/4 teaspoon salt. Cook 8 minutes, stirring. Add red potatoes, chopped, and vegetable broth. Bring to a boil, then cover and simmer. Cook 25 minutes or until potatoes are fork-tender. Remove thyme sprigs. Add asparagus, stir in navy beans, basil, and salt and pepper to taste. Can be stored for several days.*

Tahini Stuffed Sweet Potatoes

Spicy, sweet, and stuffed with tahini, these sweet potatoes will expand your horizons but not your waistline. **Calories: 402**

- **4 medium sweet potatoes**
- **1 teaspoon canola oil**
- **1 (15-oz.) can unsalted garbanzo beans, rinsed and drained**
- **2 teaspoons toasted sesame oil**
- **1 teaspoon garlic powder**
- **1/2 teaspoon kosher salt, divided**
- **1/2 teaspoon ground ginger**
- **4 tablespoons tahini**
- **1 teaspoon grated peeled fresh ginger**
- **1 teaspoon grated fresh garlic**
- **1 teaspoon rice vinegar**
- **3 tablespoons hot water**
- **4 teaspoons Sriracha chili sauce**
- **2 teaspoons water**
- **1/4 cup thinly sliced green onions**
- **1/2 teaspoon white or black sesame seeds**

Directions: *Preheat oven to 400 degrees. Rub potatoes with oil, then pierce with a fork several times on every side. Bake at 400 for one hour or until fork-tender. Cool, then split in half lengthwise.*

Toss chickpeas with sesame oil and place them on a baking sheet. Sprinkle with garlic powder, a pinch of salt, and ground ginger. Bake at 400°F for 30 minutes, stirring at least twice.

While chickpeas are baking, combine tahini, ginger, garlic, sriracha sauce and vinegar in a bowl. Add enough hot water that the paste becomes loose.

Top each sweet potato half with toasted chickpeas and tahini mix, then sprinkle with green onions and sesame seeds.

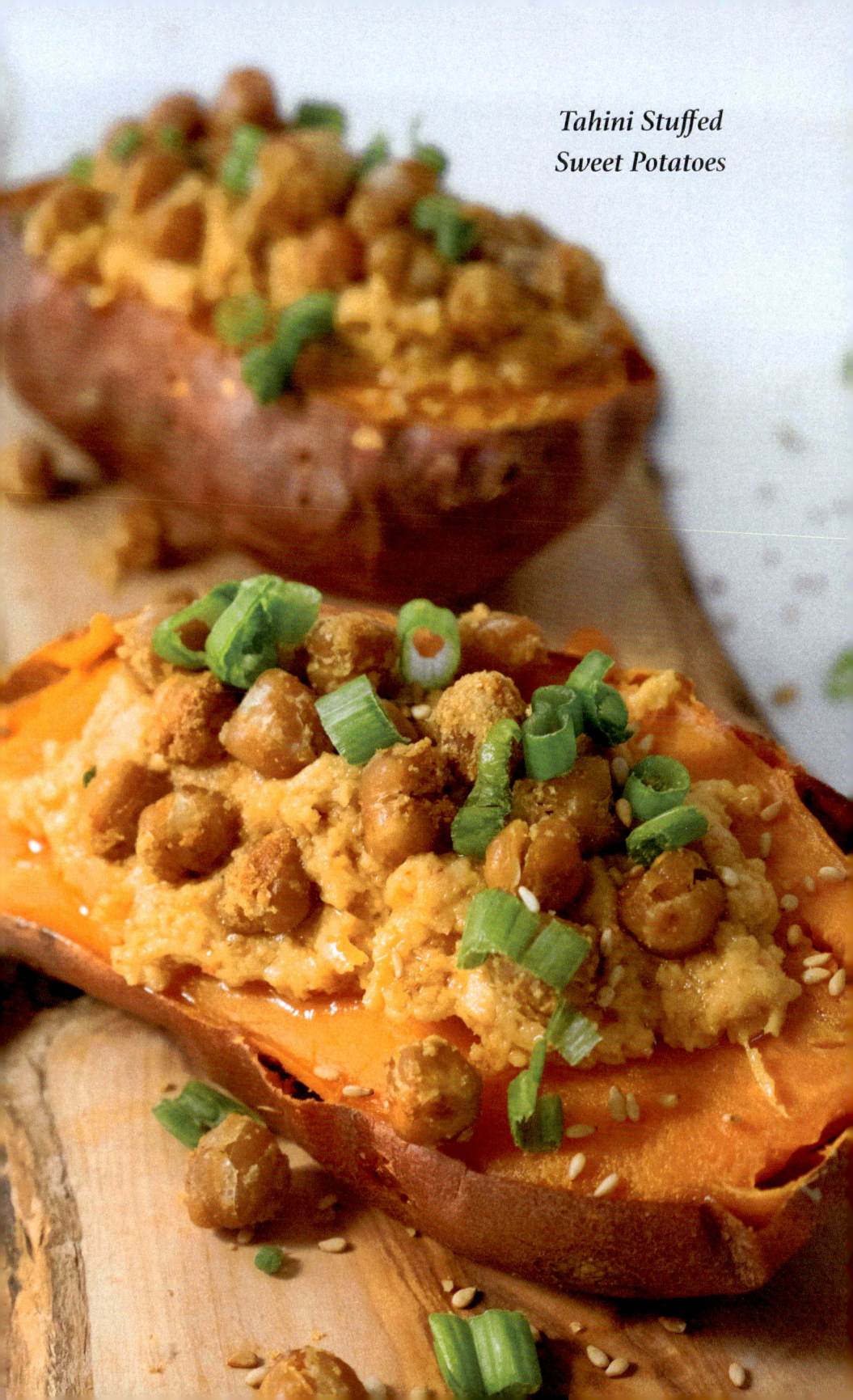

*Tahini Stuffed
Sweet Potatoes*

Grab-n-Go Dinner Options

For those evenings, when you need to get home and get dinner on the table, these grocery-store shelf solutions will do the job just fine.

Pop into Trader Joes

If you have a Trader Joes nearby, they've got some quick dinner options that'll land you in the neighborhood of where you want to be for dinner calories. Their shitake mushroom chicken, for instance, is only 180 calories per serving so you can pair it with your cucumber salad and some brown rice without worrying you'll tip the scales for daily intake.

Healthy Choice Entrees

Most grocery stores stock a variety of Healthy Choice brand entrees in the freezer section. Pick lean meats or proteins like the Cajun style chicken shrimp, which hits 220 calories per serving. Paired with some zoodles and a sprinkle of fresh parmesan, it's a wholesome choice that still feels like takeout.

Go Vegetarian with Cedar Lane

It can be difficult to find good options for the busy vegetarian. Cedar Lane has a line of both frozen and refrigerated products like paleo bowls, burritos, and tamales with a focus on nutrition and healthy ingredients. We recommend the Cedar Lane Eggplant Parm at 280 calories paired with a whole wheat baguette for dipping.

Focus on Low-Calorie-Density Foods

When you're shopping for quick dinner solutions, focus on proteins accompanied by heaping portions of vegetables. You can always choose to add small portions of grains to your meal, but the majority of your meal should be low-calorie dense foods. At 270 calories, convenient sauté and plate entrees like Bird's Eye Asian Protein Blend provide small amounts of whole grains accompanied by shelled edamame, carrots, and red peppers.

Kid-Approved Isn't as Hard as You Think

The struggle to find kid-approved, healthy dinner options is real. Don't give up, though. There are plenty of choices like Veggies Made Great Broccoli Cheddar Bake (200 calories) where the nuttiness of brown rice and the smothering of cheddar cheese hides plenty of nutrients. You can pair these with a favorite fruit and a serving of protein to round out the meal.

Save Room for Dessert

You're not full yet, are you? Good. Because we saved the stuff that will satisfy your sweet tooth for last. If you want this habit of conscious eating to become your new normal, it's critical you don't feel deprived. The Cucumber Diet is geared for weight loss, but long-term it's intended to be a paradigm shift that will mean the happy, healthy you is here to stay. It teaches you to moderate your diet so eating becomes a habit and not a hassle.

A word about fruit

Fresh fruit makes a fantastic dessert because it's usually low in calories and high in fiber, helping you digest your dinner while giving the nod to that persistent sweet tooth. However, not all fruit is created equal. Pay attention to fruits that have a high caloric cost, like bananas and mango (around 100 calories per piece), and low-calorie-density fruit like a handful of raspberries or a plum (around 20 calories).

If you've strayed outside the lines in a few spots during the day, now is the time to take up the slack with desserts under 100 calories. The recipes below range from batches of cookies you can whip up on the weekend and freeze to fruity yogurt parfaits that go easy on the extras. Decide what you have time to invest in and then go for it because you've earned a little decadence.

Keep it Simple

Greek Yogurt and Berries

Calories: 150 - *Just spoon 3.5 oz. of plain yogurt into a bowl and top with a ½ cup of berries of your choice.*

Salted Cantaloupe

Calories: 52 - *This one is so easy you'll wonder how you missed it. Take a wedge of cantaloupe (or any melon for that matter) and sprinkle with sea salt. Devour.*

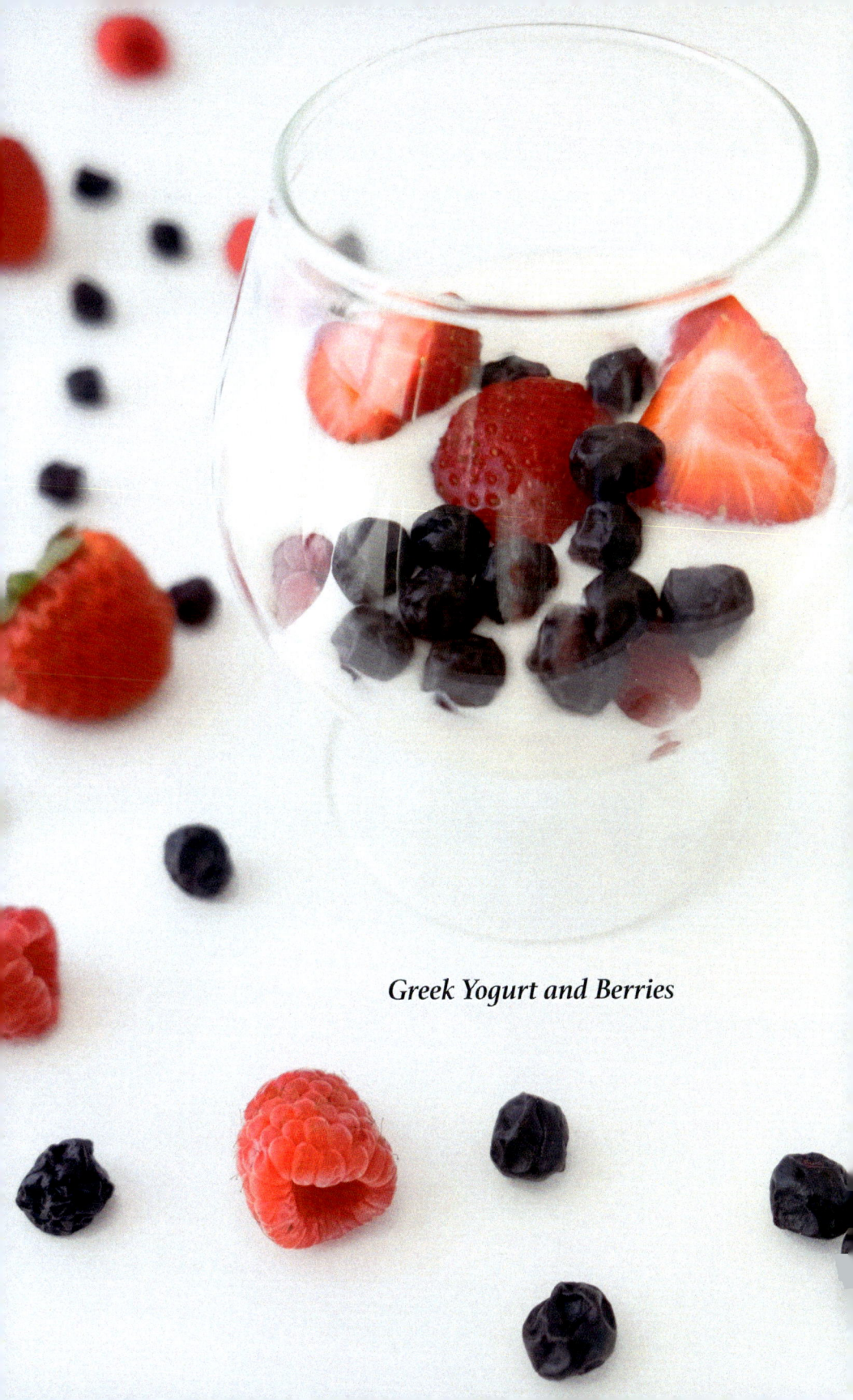

Greek Yogurt and Berries

Baked Apples

Calories: 95 - *Preheat oven to 350 degrees. Cut the top off an apple and bake in preheated oven for 30 minutes. Sprinkle with cinnamon if desired.*

Apples and Peanut or Almond Butter

Calories: 200 - *Slice a medium apple and scoop a tablespoon of peanut butter or almond butter for dipping.*

Frozen Mango Cubes

Calories: 60 - *Peel and cube mango, then freeze.*

Greek Yogurt and Honey

Calories: 80 - *This time top your 3.5 oz. of plain yogurt with a drizzle of honey for a lower calorie midnight snack.*

Cinnamon Flax Seed Pudding

Calories: 150 - *This pudding is just a blend of ½ cup cottage cheese, 1 tablespoon of flax seeds, and ½ teaspoon of cinnamon. Dig in!*

Mix-n-Match Banana Oat Cookies

The caloric count of these cookies is listed as a range because what you end up with will depend on your third ingredient. Get adventurous and see what combinations strike your fancy.

Calories: 50-80 calories per cookie (makes 16 cookies), Serving size 2-3 cookies

2 large, ripe bananas

1 3/4 cups quick oats

Choose your 3rd ingredient:

4 tablespoons peanut flour or almond butter

1/4 cup chocolate or peanut butter chips

1-2 teaspoons honey

1/4 cup cacao nibs

2 Tbsp. hazelnut spread

1/3 cup chopped nuts

1/3 cup dried fruit

1/4 cup shredded coconut

Directions: *Preheat oven to 350 degrees. Mash bananas in a bowl, then mix in oats. Gently fold in the third ingredient of your choice. Line a baking sheet with parchment paper and drop one tablespoon of dough onto the tray. Press down with the back of the spoon on the dough. Bake 15-20 minutes until firm and slightly golden. Remove and cool. Store in an airtight container.*

Oatmeal & Dark Chocolate Chunk Cookies

These satisfying cookies are an easy way to mix up some fun without going overboard on sugar and fat.

Calories: 100 per cookie (makes 24 cookies), Serving size 2 cookies

2 ounces butter (softened)

1/2 cup brown sugar

1/3 cup granulated sugar

1 large egg

1 teaspoon almond extract

1 cup all-purpose flour

1 1/2 cups old-fashioned oats, uncooked

1 teaspoon baking powder

1/2 teaspoon baking soda

1/2 teaspoon salt, plus a pinch of salt

1/4 teaspoon cardamom

1/2 cup dark chocolate chunks

Directions: *Preheat the oven to 350 degrees. Mix butter and sugar together in a stand mixer with the paddle attachment until smooth and fluffy. Add the egg and almond extract and mix thoroughly. In a separate bowl, combine the flour, oats, baking powder, baking soda, salt, and cardamom. Mix in the dry ingredients slowly on the lowest setting until just combined. Add dark chocolate chunks and stir gently.*

Drop by rounded tablespoon onto a baking sheet prepared with parchment paper, spacing about 2-inches apart. Makes 24 cookies. Bake at 350 degrees for 10-12 minutes until the edges of the cookies are slightly brown. Take cookies out, sprinkle with sea salt and let them set on the tray before removing to cooling rack. Store in airtight container.

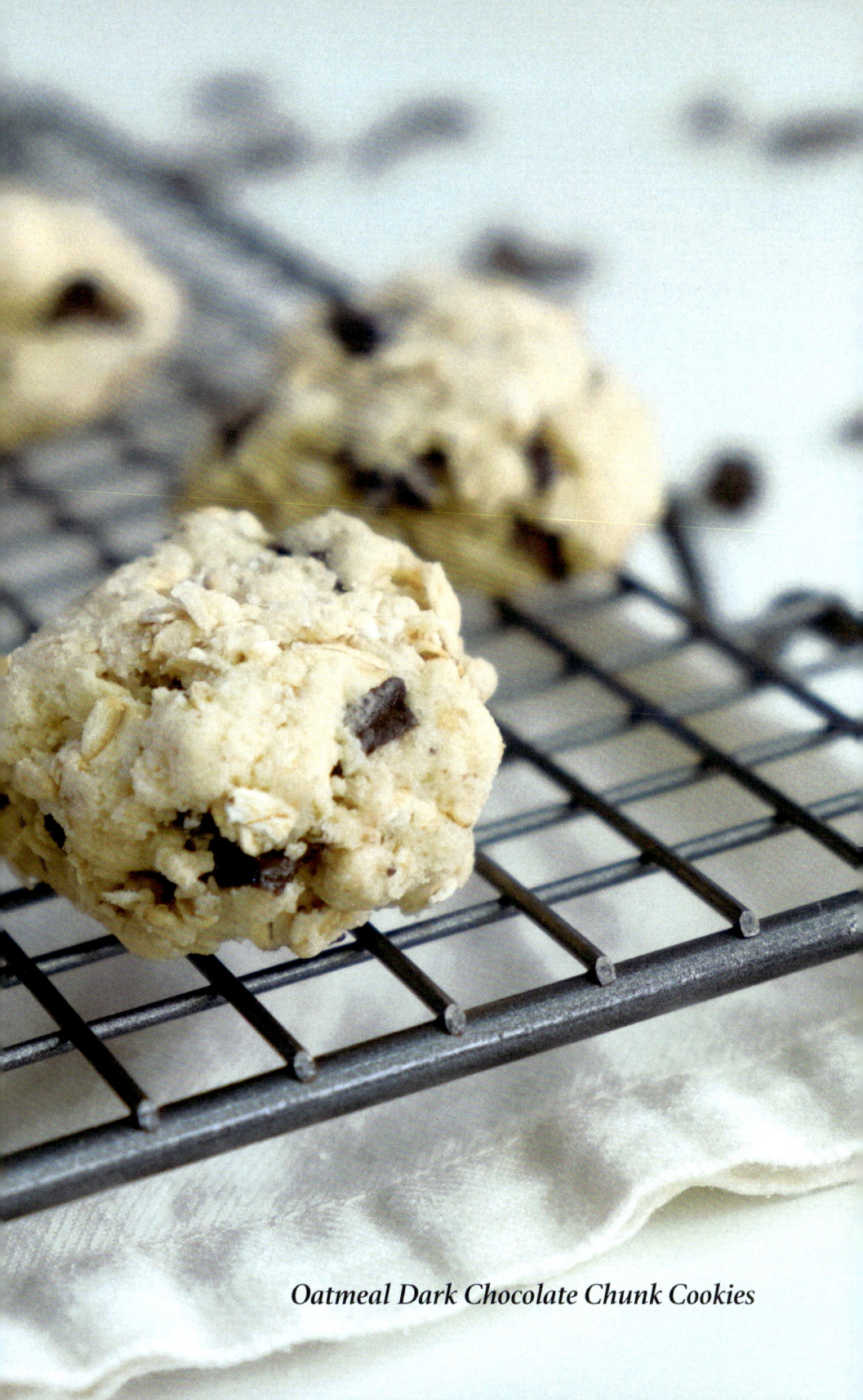

Oatmeal Dark Chocolate Chunk Cookies

Grab-n-Go Treats

These off-the-shelf desserts are for those who want a nibble of something sweet to finish the day but don't have time to turn on the oven. These little gems strike the right balance of indulgence without the side of guilt.

Coconut is Always a Good Choice

Beware the serving size, but coconut strips are a sweet treat that's packed with healthy fats. A little goes a long way though so stick with handful, which will cost you about 185 calories.

Chocolate Anyone? Yes, you can

For this diet, you're not going to have to give up your favorite indulgence. A square or two of chocolate never hurt anyone and will usually set you back about 70 calories. In fact, dark chocolate has tons of benefits in small portions, can be part of a healthy diet.

Go Light with Low-Calorie Ice Cream

It may seem trendy, but low-calorie ice cream is here to stay. Contrary to the packaging, however, you probably shouldn't devour a whole pint. But you don't have to be stingy either. At 45 calories a serving, you can definitely afford a second scoop of brands like Arctic Zero.

Look for Fiber-Forward Treats

Finding healthy dessert options doesn't have to be hard. Just look for products that have plenty of fiber and minimal additives. Figamajigs, made with figs, cocoa, and dark chocolate, fit the bill at 120 calories with 16% of your daily value of fiber.

Pay Attention to Portion Sizes

A nibble of just about anything is going to be okay as long as it slides in under your allotted calorie count. Yes, even chocolate chip cookies. For instance you can eat two of Tate's Bake Shop Chocolate Chip Cookies and still stay under 250 calories.

Dessert on a Stick

No healthy dessert compilation would be complete with Yasso's Frozen Greek Yogurt Bars. These low-calorie, high-protein treats are around 100 calories and come in tons of flavors from Butter Pecan to Mint Chocolate Chip.

A Word About Snacking

Let's be real. Snacking happens.

Snacking can sneak more calories in your daily count than you suspect. A little here and a little there definitely adds up. That's why when you begin the cucumber diet, it's best to refrain from snacking if you can. But we also recognize that sometimes even the best intentions go astray.

There isn't a caloric allocation in this diet plan for snacks, but if you need an afternoon pick me up, we have some tips. Keep in mind that if you're active and burn a few hundred calories a day, it's a little easier to make room for an extra handful of something something to tide you over until dinner.

No matter what time of day you find yourself getting the munchies, it's ideal to keep snacking to 100 – 150 calories at most. And of course, it's always best if you can eat a whole food with plenty of fiber to keep you full until your next meal.

Here are a few good options for a light afternoon snack and remember exercising portion control is critical to keeping that calorie count in range.

Salty & Savory

To keep your afternoon snack satisfying, go for salty with plenty of crunch. A focus on veggies and heart-healthy fat will give you plenty of fiber to keep you full until dinner arrives.

Grab a handful of nuts (150 calories)

It's easy to go overboard when you have a huge bag in front of you, so make each nut count. A serving of almonds is around 23 nuts or ¼ cup, while pistachios are about four calories per nut. Once you do the math, you can pop a few and get your daily dose of heart-healthy fats into the bargain.

Go for veggies and hummus (100 calories)

A modest amount of hummus goes a long way towards making humble veggies feel satisfying. Choose a serving of cucumbers, carrots, peapods, or even cherry tomatoes to dip into about two tablespoons of hummus.

Gobble some kale chips (100 calories)

Veggie-based chips are a good alternative for folks who want to feel like they're indulging in junk food but still stay on plan. You can make kale chips by tossing about 2 cups of kale with a teaspoon of olive oil and a sprinkle of salt and baking them at 400 degrees for about 8 minutes.

Get into edamame (150 calories)

Steamed soybean pods make a great snack, especially sprinkled with a little salt. You'll get lots of protein-packed into a serving size, but be sure you're eating less than a cup (about ¾ cup), so you can slide in under your calorie count for the day.

Sweet Stuff

That sweet tooth can get you into trouble, so tame into submission with these nibbles of indulgence. The secret is moderation, moderation, moderation.

Gravitate to fruit & nut butter (150 calories)

Pick a satisfying serving of fruit like a pear or apple and accompany it with a tablespoon of nut butter. You'll get a taste of both salty and sweet for the bargain of just under 150 calories.

Grab a spoon for some yogurt (100 calories)

Unadorned, yogurt is about 100 calories per serving, so you can eat a container without guilt. If you want to get more sweetness out of your snack, look for low-fat, lower-calorie options that you can combine with a few berries.

Get onboard with coconut strips (150 calories)

Coconut on its own is slightly sweet, and if you opt for unsweetened strips or chips, you can get more calorie count packed in. These are easy to overindulge in, so watch your portion size and stay under ¼ cup.

Grab dark chocolate almonds (150 calories)

There are 18 calories in every dark chocolate covered almond, so stick to a small handful that tops out at around eight almonds. Savor every morsel with the added benefits of plenty of antioxidants and iron.

Go for a handful of dried fruit (100-120 calories)

Depending on which kind you choose, a handful of dried fruit can provide fiber and a sense of fullness while still satisfying your sweet tooth. Unsweetened dried berries, apricots, and plums are typically lower in calories. You may gravitate towards fruit like mango and pineapple but be aware that they are a little higher in sugar content and thus calories.

Walk This Way

Going to the gym, spin class, running. These are all activities to include in your routine to help maintain your weight. While exercise isn't an effective weight loss strategy on its own, it's still a cornerstone of a healthy lifestyle. And if you're motivated, that's great. But a recent report from the Centers for Disease Control and Prevention says most of us are not getting enough exercise.[21]

Nationally, 18.7 percent of women and 27.2 percent of men hit the target goal considered healthy for activity in their age range. Nationally, that's an average of 22.9% or less than one-quarter of the population.[22] Some people love it, live for it, enjoy every moment. The rest of us? Not so much. Me? I can't stand it. But what I do is walk. A lot. And it makes a huge difference.

A study published in the British Journal of Sports Medicine discovered those who kept a regular walking program of 100 minutes a week or more showed significant improvements in blood pressure, slowing of resting heart rate, reduction of body fat and body weight, and reduced cholesterol.[23] They also demonstrated improved depression scores with a better quality of life and increased measures of endurance.

Walking as it turns out, is a very effective form of exercise. Take the opportunity to walk every chance you get. Don't take the elevators, take the stairs. Park in the spot furthest from the entrance at the office or the grocery store.

Better yet, go for a walk. Find a buddy who wants to go on lunch breaks or strike out on your own. Plot out a route that feels comfortable and safe. Know where you're going, and you'll feel more comfortable and less likely to bug out or feel self-conscious. You don't even need a fancy wearable fitness device, although they can be fun to encourage a little healthy competition among friends. Most smartphones track your steps for you, if not, there are lots of apps for that as well.

I start every weekday with a 45 minute to one-hour walk. I get up, put on sweats, and go. Sometimes I walk with a friend. Sometimes I walk alone. If I'm alone, I put on earphones and tune out. Start looking at your steps and making targets. Every step counts. Two thousand steps is a mile. A mile is 100 calories. It all adds up. And the benefit of burning those calories means you'll have more bandwidth to spend on your daily caloric allocation.

It's also worth noting that while exercise isn't effective as a weight-loss strategy by itself, it can be a critical part of maintaining your weight over time. Once you've reached your target goal, you're going to start feeling great. And it'll be tempting to let some junk sneak back into your life. Keeping a consistent, exercise regime doing something you enjoy will keep you motivated and prevent weight gain from creeping up on you.

Change your Mindset – Change your Life!

Now that you've read the book, it should be obvious why just dieting all the time, going from diet to diet, doesn't work. It's unhealthy and emotionally draining. When you use dieting as a constant fallback, it's like giving yourself permission to overeat. That's not only yo-yo dieting, it's an emotional roller coaster ride as well.

When we eat unconsciously, we too often end up feeling guilty. "I shouldn't eat this... I can't believe I ate that... I feel awful... Oh well, I'll start that diet Monday." That's a conversation many of us are all too familiar with. And it's emotionally exhausting. That's no way to live. But YOU have to power to change it.

Too many diet plans want you to eat their food, or they use some alternate method of keeping you dependent upon their plan. They would like you to believe that you are not capable or trustworthy to make your own choices. "It's too hard, don't bother, we can do it for you." Most plans are simply a crutch to help you lose weight. Then what?

In most of these cases, there's nothing conscious about short-term weight loss. And without their diet-plan crutch, it's difficult to truly sustain or manage your weight long term. The Cucumber Diet is different. Instead of giving you a crutch, we teach you the tenets of conscious eating. A few simple tools that allow you to manage your weight logically. Managing your weight logically can be as simple a task as going to the supermarket – you know what you have to spend, just stay within your budget. The only difference is thinking calories in place of dollars.

Many diet programs would have you believe that knowing your caloric intake is like being "a slave to calories". But that's not true. No truer than saying that going to the grocery store and not knowing the price of what you buy makes you "a slave to dollars". And as we've demonstrated earlier, eating consciously is not as hard as many diet plans would have you believe. Because conscious eating is a way of managing your weight logically, and once you begin the practice, managing your weight becomes innate. You're not counting calories all day, you're simply conscious of where you're at for the day. That's a lot more conscious than having absolutely no idea.

Of course, there are no absolutes. It's unlikely that anyone is going to eat whole foods exclusively. You're going to want an occasional processed chip. Simply make whole foods the mainstay of your diet and eat the high calorie density foods, like chips, more judiciously.

Remember, you only need to diet if you're not managing your weight. And with conscious eating, you can manage your weight easily, logically, healthfully and eliminate the guilt and stress of yo-yo dieting.

Once more for Those in the Back

The power of conscious eating is real. And now that you've read the book, you're armed with some solid tools to implement conscious eating into your life. And of course awareness is half the battle! If your goal is to lose weight, eat healthy, feel satisfied and learn to moderate your weight, you can achieve it all with the cucumber diet.

In this final chapter, we're going to recap the basics of the plan and lay out a few additional tips to get you going and keep you on track. But first, let's talk about the topic that everybody is thinking about and nobody wants to talk about - weight. I'll start with mine.

People who know me would say, "you don't need to lose weight"—that's true for me now, though it wasn't always. But for me, it's not about how much I weigh. It's about how I feel—both how I feel physically and how I feel about myself. I believe the right weight is the one at which you feel comfortable and happy, regardless of standards or sizes.

We're all different, with various body types, and living to meet the standards of others is, in my opinion, not living well. So, if you're happy at a given weight, that's the right weight for you. So don't sweat it! Your weight is whatever makes you happy – not everyone else. The only caveat to this is that you're healthy, so if your doctor thinks your weight is unhealthy you should heed their advice.

Probably, though, if you are reading this, you would feel happier at a different weight, and the cucumber diet can help get you there. And I promise you will be happier when you are eating consciously, thinking about what you eat in a positive, constructive and self-confident way, not with guilt or pain. Conscious eating makes every day happier and better.

Empower Yourself!

There's a certain kind of satisfaction that comes from knowing I don't have to worry about my weight. That I can eat well and moderate my weight naturally. I know what weight I feel good at, and I simply keep it there. I don't let food run me. I simply practice conscious eating. Once I learned to do it, I was surprised it became innate to me so quickly.

And in way, it's sort of fun, like a numbers game. Not so different from tracking your steps or going shopping. I know my caloric intake and stay within my personal range without much thought. I love food, eat well and maintain my weight with ease.

You can do it too. When you start the cucumber diet and embrace conscious eating, you will be surprised at how easy and even fun it is, and you will love the feeling it gives you when you replace negative eating habits and negative thoughts with positive and constructive ones.

Conscious eating makes it simple. It's almost impossible to image that I had such little awareness of what I was eating before. Counting calories works. We use math in almost every aspect of our lives and it's a superb tool, not a burden.

Let these three basic tenets be your guide:

Which Kinds Of Foods Are You Eating?

Eat more whole foods. Low calorie density foods are filling, that's more food for less calories.

How Much Are You Eating?

Measure what a serving size is. You'll learn fast when you see what a true serving size looks like.

What's The Caloric Cost Of What You're Eating?

Knowing the number of calories in food is quite easy. An average egg will always be 78 calories, and a large cucumber 45 calories. It's not as many items as it seems. There's a handy calorie reference guide in the back of the book.

These are really very easy and logical steps. Conscious eating is about being aware. Know what you're eating, and you can moderate your caloric intake and resulting weight naturally. Aside from the three basic tenets of the Cucumber Diet, here are a few good tips that are easy to remember and will help keep you on track.

Put Down the Fork

Put down the damn fork. If you just think about that, you'll start to catch yourself efficiently shoveling food. That doesn't add to your enjoyment of food, it just adds to your calories. When you become conscious of how you are eating, putting down your fork will occur naturally. In the meantime, simply put your fork down on the table after every bite. Make it a habit. Take your time. Allow your stomach to tell your brain you're full. That takes about 20 minutes. So, if you eat in 10 or 15 minutes you won't feel full until well after you've consumed much more than you intended. This also holds true if you're eating a sandwich, wrap or something that doesn't require a fork. Take a bite and give it a rest. The point is the same - to slow yourself down.

It's Okay Not to Finish

This one is super important. It's okay not to finish. Our instinct is to clean the plate. In fact, most of us were taught to eat that way. But why? Being stuffed or full doesn't even feel good. Simply having awareness about that is what conscious eating is about. When you get to the point where you feel satisfied, stop eating even if there's still some food on the plate. It really is okay not to finish.

Extra Credit – Walk This Way

Walking equals big bonus points. It's excellent exercise, doesn't require equipment or a designated time. Walk anywhere and everywhere you can. It's not only good for you but it can knock quite a few calories off and help you lose weight. Start really looking at your daily steps. Every step counts. Two thousand steps are a mile. A mile is 100 calories. It adds up and you'll feel better knowing you're burning those calories and staying within your daily caloric allocation.

Now you know.

For decades we've been told a litany of facts about eating that were a confusing mess. I have come to recognize that it wasn't my fault that I didn't know how to eat, and it's not your fault either. But now we know. It's not about processed foods packed with sugar and chemicals. It's about whole foods and eating well. Embracing nutritious whole foods that taste great, are satisfying and help you manage your weight.

You're likely never going to eat one hundred percent whole foods, that's okay. Don't deny yourself an occasional chip or cookie – it's not an all or nothing proposition and you'll never win by depriving yourself of something you really want. But you are now empowered with an eating superpower – awareness. You are armed with awareness and with the power of conscious eating. You have the cucumber diet and its three simple tenets. You are ready to win at this game of eating well and taking care of you.

Now that you have the power, you could do this alone. But what's the fun in that?

The Cucumber Diet Community

Ask questions, share your personal experiences and connect with others on our official Twitter page @TheCucumberDiet We will offer some support as well as regular updates on new recipes and more. Hope to see you there!

Quick Reference Calorie Guide

Ingredient	Serving	Calories
Veggies		
Celery	2 stalks	14
Mushrooms	½ cup	19
Spinach	4 cups	20
Yellow squash	½ cup	20
Eggplant	½ cup or 3 slices	20
Zucchini	¾ cup	21
Tomatoes	½ cup	22
Bell Peppers	½ cup	25
Broccoli	1 cup	29
Cauliflower	1 cup	29
Asparagus	½ cup	29
Sundried tomatoes	2 pieces	30
Carrots	½ cup or 1 medium carrot	38
Roasted red pepper	1 pepper	50
Kale	2 cups	53
Leek	1 leek	54
Onion	1 medium onion	56
Green peas	½ cup	78
Sweet Potatoes	1 cup	130
Potatoes	1 cup	220
Avocado	2 Tbsp	167
Fruits		
Plums	1 medium	30
Strawberries	1 cup	36
Peaches	1 medium	41
Blueberries	1 cup	50
Cantaloupe	1 cup	54
Raspberries	1 cup	57
Banana	1 medium	88
Apple	1 medium	94
Orange juice	1 cup	111
Mango	1 medium	124
Raisins	¼ cup or 1 snack box	140
Applesauce	1 cup	156
Dried fruit	½ cup	275

Ingredient	Serving	Calories

Protein/Meat

Ingredient	Serving	Calories
Sesame seeds	1 Tbsp	45
Chia seeds	1 Tbsp	60
Cooked Ham	3 slices	70
Eggs	1 large egg	71
Bacon	1 slice	80
Navy beans	¼ cup	90
Peanut butter	1 Tbsp.	95
Cashew butter	1 Tbsp.	97
Almond butter	1 Tbsp.	98
Kidney beans	½ cup	100
Trout	1 medium filet, no skin	108
Garbanzo beans (chickpeas)	½ cup	110
Edamame	½ cup, shelled	110
Tilapia	1 medium filet, no skin	111
Smoked Turkey	3 slices	125
Flax seeds	2 Tbsp.	130
Pork Tenderloin	4 oz.	130
Black-eyed peas	¼ cup	140
Black beans	¼ cup	150
Shrimp	1 cup shelled & cooked	160
Cashews	¼ cup	160
Pistachios	¼ cup, shelled	160
Almonds	¼ cup	170
Pumpkin seeds	¼ cup, shelled and raw	180
Tahini	1 Tbsp.	180
Flank steak	4 oz.	186
Sirloin steak	4 oz.	195
Chicken breast	1 medium breast, no skin	210
Hazelnut spread	2 Tbsp.	210
Salmon	1 medium filet, no skin	211
Ground turkey	4 oz., cooked	230

Ingredient	Serving	Calories

Dairy

Ingredient	Serving	Calories
Feta cheese	2 Tbsp., crumbled	44
Parmesan cheese	2 Tbsp., grated	56
Coconut milk	1 cup	75
Skim milk	1 cup	79
Mozzarella cheese	¼ cup, grated	80
Cheddar cheese	1 slice	84
Almond milk	1 cup	89
Heavy cream	2 Tbsp.	100
Butter	1 Tbsp.	100
Blue cheese	2 Tbsp.	100
Smoked gouda cheese	1 slice	110
Greek yogurt	½ cup	160

Grains

Ingredient	Serving	Calories
Breadcrumbs	¼ cup	70
Coconut flour	2 Tbsp.	70
White, all-purpose flour	¼ cup	110
Quinoa	½ cup, cooked	111
Whole-wheat hamburger bun	1 bun	120
Fiber Cereal	1 cup	124
Whole-wheat tortilla	1 large tortilla	130
Whole-wheat baguette	3, 1-inch slices	130
Whole-wheat bread	1 slice, sandwich loaf	140
Granola	¼ cup	146
Tortilla chips	15 chips	150
Quick oats	½ cup, cooked	150
Couscous	½ cup, cooked	150
Arborio rice	¾ cup, cooked	154
Pita bread	1 medium pita	157
Brown rice	¾ cup, cooked	190
Whole-wheat pasta	½ cup	200

Ingredient	Serving	Calories

Fats & Sugars

Ingredient	Serving	Calories
Sugar, white	1 Tbsp.	15
Sugar, brown	1 Tbsp.	17
Maple syrup	1 Tbsp.	52
Honey	1 Tbsp.	63
Dark Chocolate	1 square inch	95
Olive oil	1 Tbsp.	119
Sesame oil	1 Tbsp.	120
Coconut oil	1 Tbsp.	121
Shredded coconut	¼ cup	130

* Calorie values provided courtesy of the USDA Food Database